LEARNING
TO LIVE WITH
HYPERTENSION

A MIPI Publication

CONSULTANTS

Aram V. Chobanian, M.D., Director, Cardiovascular Institute and Professor of Medicine, Boston University School of Medicine, Boston, Massachusetts

Sue B. Foster, R.N., M.S.N., Director, Nursing Education and Research Program, Beth Israel Hospital, Boston, Massachusetts

John Jainchill, M.D., Internist, The Urban Medical Group, Inc.; Assistant Professor of Socio-Medical Sciences, Boston University School of Medicine, Boston, Massachusetts

Lawrence R. Krakoff, M.D., Professor of Medicine and Chief, Hypertension Division, Mount Sinai School of Medicine of the City University of New York, New York, New York

James O. Taylor, M.D., Medical Director, East Boston Neighborhood Health Center; Associate Clinical Professor of Medicine, Brigham and Women's Hospital and Harvard Medical School, Boston, Massachusetts

PATIENT ADVISERS

Mary Claire Adams   John R. Bailey   Laura Carlson   Calvin Clemons   Azell Davis   Barbara Droz

SERIES ADVISORY COMMITTEE

Pamela W. Brown, R.N., M.S., Assistant Professor of Nursing, Massachusetts College of Pharmacy and Allied Health Sciences, Boston, Massachusetts

Ralph Hingson, Sc.D., Associate Professor of Socio-Medical Sciences, Boston University Schools of Medicine and Public Health, Boston, Massachusetts

John D. Stoeckle, M.D., Professor of Medicine, Harvard Medical School, and Physician, Massachusetts General Hospital, Boston, Massachusetts

SERIES STAFF

Directors: Judith P. Swazey, Ph.D., President, Acadia Institute, Bar Harbor, Maine; Board of Directors, Medicine In the Public Interest.

Louis Lasagna, M.D., Academic Dean, School of Medicine, and Dean, Sackler School of Graduate Biomedical Science, Tufts University, Boston, Massachusetts; President, Board of Directors, Medicine In the Public Interest.

Robert J. Levine, M.D., Professor of Medicine, Lecturer in Pharmacology, Yale University School of Medicine, New Haven, Connecticut; Board of Directors, Medicine In the Public Interest.

Writer and Editor: Cynthia B. Wong

Researcher: Judith C. Watkins

TABLE OF CONTENTS

TO THE READER

Learning to Live with Hypertension is one in a series of books prepared for patients by Medicine in the Public Interest, Inc. The purpose of this book is to provide medically accurate and readily understandable information about the nature and treatment of hypertension and to suggest ways in which you may be better able to cope with it.

In preparing the book, we worked closely with doctors, nurses, and other medical specialists in the field of hypertension, as well as with people who are living with the condition. The professional advisers have the technical expertise regarding what patients *ought* to know, while the patient advisers helped us with what patients *want* to know and how it feels to live with hypertension.

One of our goals in this book is to improve the communication between you and those who are involved in your medical care. We hope that you and they—and your family—will use it together.

Learning to Live with Hypertension contains information for patients that can be helpful in treating hypertension. This information is not intended to replace the advice of a doctor.

No two cases of hypertension are alike. Your doctor has chosen a treatment program that is specific to your individual needs. To get the most benefit from your program, keep your doctor fully informed of your progress.

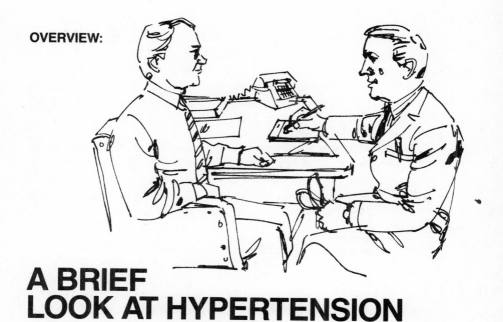

A BRIEF LOOK AT HYPERTENSION

What is hypertension?

How does it happen?

Why me?

How will it affect my daily life?

If you have recently been told that you have hypertension (also called *high blood pressure*), or even if you have had it for some time, these are probably some of the questions you have been asking. As time goes on, you will have others. In this book, we hope to encourage you to ask, to find out how you can help manage your high blood pressure and be an active partner in taking care of your health. We want to help you understand hypertension, but our emphasis is on *living* with it.

Although treatment for high blood pressure is fairly simple, as you will see, the condition itself is quite complex. Even the experts don't know all there is to know about it. Certainly, nobody expects you to learn it all at once. You may not understand everything that the doctor has told you so far. You may want to know more but may be anxious about what you would learn. You may not even know what questions to ask.

But you probably do want to know, quickly, what it really means and how it will affect your daily life. Therefore, as a way of introducing you to hypertension, we begin here with a brief picture, to give you an overview in a few pages. Then later—perhaps much later—as questions come up and as you are ready to learn more about a particular subject, we hope that you will read on.

In summary, this book is *your* guide, to be used in whatever way you find helpful—to learn, to raise questions, or to use as a reference. And, as you read this, we encourage you to talk about it and use it together with your doctor, your family, and others involved in your care.

> Fortunately, I can ask the people at the clinic anything. They always take the time to talk to me and listen to my problems.
> —Louise M.

In living with hypertension, you will probably work with many people. Your primary contact will usually be your doctor. But nurses, physician's assistants, dietitians, pharmacists and many other specialists also play important roles. Please keep in mind, as you use this book, that these other individuals are also included when we refer to "your doctor."

WHAT IS HYPERTENSION?

Blood is constantly circulating throughout your body under pressure. It travels through a network of blood vessels called *veins* and *arteries*. Your heart works like a pump, forcing blood out into the arteries with every beat. The arteries deliver the blood, which contains oxygen and other nourishment, to all the cells and tissues in your body. Then the blood returns to your heart through the veins. Your heart and blood vessels work closely together, making up your *circulatory system*.

As blood travels through your arteries, it pushes against their walls. The force of the blood against the artery walls is called *blood pressure*. Your blood pressure changes often—during the day and from one day to another—depending on your activities and how you feel. Also, different parts of your body need more blood at certain times. A complex control system regulates the delivery of blood throughout your body and usually keeps the pressure within a certain range.

While everybody's blood pressure rises and falls, the condition called high blood pressure exists when your blood pressure is *consistently* higher than normal. Doctors call this *hypertension*, which means there is *too much* (hyper-) *force* or tension on the artery walls. It does *not* mean nervousness. Many relaxed and easygoing people have hypertension.

WHY IS HIGH BLOOD PRESSURE A PROBLEM?

> If you haven't got it, you don't even think about it. Oh, I knew high blood pressure *could* be a problem, but I wasn't really worried about it. I was much more concerned about cancer.
> —Debra S.

Usually, high blood pressure produces no symptoms. In fact, you probably feel fine, so it's easy to wonder what all the fuss is about. Indeed, hypertension is not usually a problem if it is treated and brought under control. The problem comes if it is *not* treated. Untreated, blood pressure will just go higher. And this can lead to some very serious complications, including heart attacks and strokes. High blood pressure is one of the most important *risk factors* for developing a serious heart or blood vessel disease. Thus, the main reason for treating high blood pressure is to *prevent* you from becoming ill. Studies have shown that the serious effects can usually be prevented when blood pressure is brought down and kept under control.

Still, this silent condition presents a major health problem in this country. For example:
- It is estimated that half of all Americans will develop hypertension at some time in their lives.
- Millions of people who have high blood pressure—perhaps as many as one-third of them—don't know it.
- About 25 percent of those who are being treated do not have their blood pressure under control.
- People with high blood pressure are five times more likely to have a heart attack than people whose blood pressure is normal, and 90 percent of all stroke victims have high blood pressure.

Let's look at some of the reasons for these numbers. Even though high blood pressure is very common, many people do not understand what it is and what it does. Several misconceptions surround it. One, as we said, is the word hypertension itself. Many people think that only people who are tense and nervous can get it.

Therefore, some people who have been told that they have hypertension don't really believe it. Or they may follow their treatment program only when they feel tense.

Another false belief is that hypertension affects only the elderly. This is not true. And still other people believe that high blood pressure always produces symptoms. Therefore, people who feel OK may not bother to have their blood pressure checked regularly. They may have high blood pressure and not know it. High blood pressure seldom gives warning signs. The only way to diagnose it is from a series of blood pressure measurements. Because it has no symptoms, high blood pressure may exist for years unless it is found in a routine checkup.

Similarly, some people who have been told that they have high blood pressure don't seek treatment or stop treatment because they feel fine. Or they take their pills only when they think that their pressure is up. You cannot tell when your pressure is up without measuring it. People who are taking medicine for hypertension need to take it regularly, regardless of how they feel.

In the last several years, because of national campaigns and public information programs, many more millions of people have been diagnosed and treated. There have also been medical improvements in the treatment and control of high blood pressure. And people have been making other healthy lifestyle changes. As a result, the death rate from high blood pressure and related diseases has dropped 35 percent in the last 10 years or so. This news has encouraged further efforts to educate the public.

> I found out about my high blood pressure when a worker from a screening program came to my door. The program is one of the most important things that ever happened to me.
> —Paul W.

TREATMENT FOR HIGH BLOOD PRESSURE

Unfortunately, nobody really knows what causes high blood pressure. In at least 9 out of 10 cases, no cause can be found. For these *there is no cure*. However, in almost every case, hypertension can be *controlled*. Treatment today is very successful.

The main form of treatment for hypertension is through drugs, and there are many kinds available. *Diuretic* drugs are the most common. They wash excess fluid and salt from your body and relieve the pressure on the arteries. If a diuretic alone does not lower your blood pressure enough, other drugs may be prescribed instead of or in addition to the diuretic.

All medicines may have unintended actions on the body. These are called side effects. They are usually mild and may not even be noticed. They often go away after your body gets used to the drug. Occasionally, however, side effects continue and cause people to stop taking the medicine. In almost every case, the side effects can be removed by trying a different drug, a lower dosage, or some other drug that offsets them. In other words, something can usually be done about any side effect that you might have. But it's up to you to let your doctor know if a problem occurs.

Most people will need to take drugs, but blood pressure can sometimes be controlled by other means. Some people may benefit by exercising, losing weight, and eating less salt, or learning how to relax. If the blood pressure is only slightly high, these measures may be enough to bring it down to normal. In other cases, these forms of therapy may mean fewer drugs or lower dosages.

TAKING IT SERIOUSLY

We want to emphasize that high blood pressure is usually a problem only when it is *not* treated and kept under control. Unfortunately, some people don't take it seriously and never follow through with their treatment program. Others stop treatment after bringing their pressure down, thinking that they are cured.

One of the hardest things to understand is that treatment is a lifelong project. Blood pressure can almost always be lowered. But if you don't keep it under control once you have brought it down, it will just go right back up again. This idea can seem discouraging at first, but the sooner you start treatment and settle into a routine, the easier it will be.

SETTLING INTO A ROUTINE

There are two major goals in treating high blood pressure. The first—and most important one—is to lower your blood pressure and to keep it down. The second goal is to do it as comfortably as possible. For most people, these goals are met with one or two drugs and perhaps some dietary changes. For everybody, there's an answer. Most people do not have to make major changes in their style of living.

> I don't consider myself sick. I do everything I've always done, except that now I take pills. —Louise M.

The early stage may be the most difficult, as you adjust to the fact that you have a medical condition that needs treatment and as you and your doctor find out what treatment program works best for you. But after that, things should settle into a fairly easy routine.

> My mother has been on medication for hypertension for 30 years and is still alive at 81. Since my pressure is now being controlled, I'm not worried. —Nancy L.

Understanding what hypertension is, recognizing that there are things that you can do that will make a difference, and having confidence in yourself and your doctor are important parts of living well with high blood pressure.

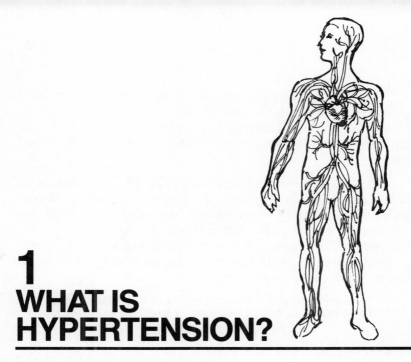

1
WHAT IS HYPERTENSION?

YOUR HEART AND CIRCULATION

Most people know very little about one of the world's hardest working and most efficient pumps—the heart—and the miles of blood vessels that circulate blood throughout the body. If you, like millions of other people, are living with high blood pressure, then learning about your heart and circulation may help you see why it's important to take good care of yourself, your heart, and your high blood pressure.

Your Heart

Your heart is a hollow organ, about the size of a large fist, with a very tough muscular wall called the *myocardium* ("myo-" means "muscle," and "cardium" means "heart"). It is shaped somewhat like an eggplant and weighs between 7 and 12 ounces. Lying in the center of your chest behind the breastbone, your heart is protected by your rib cage and by a strong covering of tissue.

Your Blood Vessels

As your heart beats, it pumps blood and nourishment through a system of *blood vessels*, elastic-like tubes that carry blood to every part of your body and back to your heart. Your heart and blood vessels make up your *cardiovascular system* ("vascular" means "vessels") or, more simply, your *circulatory system*.

Blood flows away from the heart in *arteries* and returns to it in *veins*. The blood vessels close to your heart are large, about as thick as your thumb. Then, as they go to different parts of your body, they branch off like a tree into smaller and smaller limbs and twigs.

The smallest arteries are called *arterioles*, which then subdivide into tiny *capillaries*. The capillaries wind in and out among all your body's cells, delivering nutrients and oxygen through their thin walls directly to the cells around them. At the same time, the capillaries pick up carbon dioxide and other waste products from the cells and pass them to the smallest veins, which lead to larger veins, and so on, back to your heart.

> They've told me a lot at the clinic, but I never did understand how blood goes through the body until now.   —Louise M.

Your Very Special Pump

The vast network of blood vessels in your body is about 70,000 miles long! Your heart beats about 70 times a minute, or about 100,000 times a day, and pumps the same 8 to 12 pints of blood throughout your circulatory system over and over again. Releasing 2 to 3 ounces of blood with each beat, your heart pumps the equivalent of about 2000 gallons a day.

How does your heart do all this work? Your heart is a simple muscular machine, much like a pump. The work is done by the myocardium, the heart's tough muscular wall. When your heart muscle tightens up, or *contracts*, blood is forced out of your heart and sent on its way throughout your body. Then your heart relaxes and fills up with fresh blood. This pumping action is similar to a bulb syringe or a turkey baster; when you squeeze the bulb of the baster, turkey juices are forced out.

Actually, your heart is a double pump (a right pump and a left pump) and works closely with your lungs. Each side of the heart has two chambers, an *atrium* and a *ventricle*. After your cells have taken up the oxygen and other nutrients from the blood, that blood returns from all over your body through veins into your right atrium and then into the right ventricle. As the ventricle contracts, the blood is pumped into both lungs, where carbon dioxide is released and fresh oxygen absorbed as you breathe. The fresh blood then flows into the left atrium, passes into the left ventricle, and is pumped out into the arteries, to be delivered again to your cells. And on it goes, making well over 1000 round trips a day.

The two sides of your heart, of course, work at the same time. Blood is always filling both sides. The two atria contract at the same time, sending blood into the ventricles. Then, as the atria relax, the ventricles contract, forcing blood out to the lungs and the body. A series of valves in the veins open and close with your heartbeat, keeping the blood flowing in one direction and preventing it from backing up.

Your Blood Pressure

As blood circulates through your body, it pushes against the walls of your arteries. The arteries stretch and contract as the blood pulses through. Every time your heart contracts, the pressure on the arteries increases; when your heart relaxes, the pressure goes down. Your *blood pressure* is a measure of the force of your blood against your artery walls.

At any one moment, your blood pressure depends on several things. First, everybody's blood pressure rises and falls many times in the course of the day and from day to day. A lot depends on what you are doing or how you feel. Blood pressure increases when you are anxious, upset, or afraid, and it decreases when the stressful situation is over. It also rises when you exercise and falls when you rest.

Also, the *demand* for blood from different parts of your body varies. For example, when you run, your leg muscles need more blood than usual. In response, your heart and arteries automatically send more blood and oxygen to those muscles.

Your Blood Pressure Control System

A complex system controls and regulates your blood pressure. Without such a control system, for instance, all the blood would rush to your feet whenever you stood up, your pressure would fall, and you would faint. Your kidneys, brain, and nervous system play a large part in regulating the pressure. In different ways, they raise and lower the pressure in response to the varying demands of your body for blood. The control system also acts to keep your blood pressure within a certain "preset" range. The system senses when the pressure is too high or too low and makes whatever adjustments are necessary by releasing chemical substances called *hormones*.

Your blood pressure also depends on other factors:

- Your heart muscle's strength and ability to pump blood.
- The volume of blood in circulation.
- The general condition of your arteries, which have several jobs. They smooth out the spurts of blood pumped by your heart, delivering the blood in a steady flow to all areas of your body. Then the smallest arteries (the arterioles) make sure that whatever part of the body needs more blood at the moment gets it. They do this by changing their width. For example, by contracting, or tightening up, the arterioles provide resistance to the flow of blood. The resistance limits the volume of blood to one area so that another area can get more.

> What a fascinating thought that the arteries have such power.
> —Nancy L.

All these mechanisms work automatically and at the same time, usually making tiny adjustments to produce the right blood pressure for the occasion. However, if something goes wrong with any of the control mechanisms—for example, if a signal in the central nervous system is faulty—the result may be *high blood pressure*, or *hypertension*.

HYPERTENSION

As we have seen, blood pressure goes up and down throughout the day. So, in a way, we may all have "high" blood pressure several times a day and normal pressure at other times. These occasional ups and downs are not usually a problem. The body's control system generally takes care of them. The problem comes when blood pressure is consistently higher than it should be, when the pressure is too high too often.

Doctors define *hypertension*, or high blood pressure, as a *medical condition in which several blood pressure readings show a pattern of high pressure*. The "tension" in the word "hypertension" refers to the tension or pressure on the artery walls, and "hyper" means "too much." Unfortunately, the word itself leads to confusion. Many people believe that hypertension means tenseness or nervousness and that only nervous or tense people can get it. But, in fact, anybody can get it. A great many people with high blood pressure are calm and easygoing.

Hypertension is diagnosed by taking a series of blood pressure readings several days or weeks apart. Unless the pressure is extremely high, a single reading is not usually enough, because the pressure changes from day to day. Your pressure may even be higher in the doctor's office than at home simply because you may not be relaxed. Therefore, several readings over time are necessary to establish a *pattern* of high blood pressure.

Blood pressure readings have two numbers, such as 140/90, which is said aloud as "one-forty over ninety." Pressure is measured in *millimeters (mm) of mercury (Hg)*. The first number is the *systolic pressure*. This is the pressure of the blood against the artery walls as it is forced out of the heart. The systolic pressure is the maximum pressure on the arteries. The second number is the *diastolic pressure*, which is the pressure on the artery walls when the heart is at rest between beats. It is also a measure of the resting pressure of the system.

Actually, doctors don't agree on an exact number above which blood pressure may be dangerous and below which it is O K. Furthermore, in diagnosing high blood pressure for any one individual, doctors usually consider other factors about the person. These factors include age, other medical conditions or medicines, and the presence of other risk factors for heart disease.

Although they may not agree on when blood pressure is "too high," doctors do agree that some number is needed for comparison. Today, most doctors accept 120/80 mm Hg as the common normal pressure for adults, although some lower numbers and values up to 140/90 mm Hg are included in the normal range. *Blood pressure of 140/90 mm Hg or above is usually considered high.*

Classifications of High Blood Pressure

Either systolic pressure or diastolic pressure, or both, may be high. A systolic pressure of 140 mm Hg or higher is considered too high. But for diagnosing and treating high blood pressure, doctors generally use the diastolic pressure, the pressure when your heart is relaxed. Therefore, *high blood pressure is usually classified according to the diastolic pressure*, as follows:

- **Normal blood pressure:** diastolic pressure below 90 mm Hg.
- **Mild hypertension:** diastolic pressure between 90 and 104 mm Hg.
- **Moderate hypertension:** diastolic pressure between 105 and 114 mm Hg.

- **Severe hypertension:** diastolic pressure of 115 mm Hg or more.

About 70 percent of those whose pressure is too high have mild hypertension. Another 20 percent have moderate hypertension, and about 10 percent have severe hypertension.

> "Mild" doesn't mean that you can ignore it. Even people with mild hypertension will benefit a great deal by learning about and controlling high blood pressure. —Dr. W.

Two other kinds of high blood pressure should be mentioned. A severe, rapidly progressive—but rare—form of high blood pressure is called *accelerated* or *malignant hypertension*. Here, the diastolic pressure is extremely high—130 mm Hg or more (the systolic pressure is usually well into the 200s). Malignant hypertension (which has no relation to cancer) is a crisis condition and causes a great deal of damage to various organs in the body. If it is not treated, death may occur within months.

Some people have borderline or *labile hypertension* (also called *transient hypertension*). Labile hypertension exists when someone has occasional high readings, often when under stress. Actually, everyone's blood pressure is labile (likely to change), but the term "labile hypertension" refers to people whose blood pressure is usually normal but occasionally above normal. About 10 to 25 percent of those with labile hypertension eventually progress to mild hypertension.

Very Few Symptoms

Although high blood pressure is easy to diagnose, it often goes undiscovered for years unless it is found in a routine blood pressure reading or physical examination. Hypertension seldom gives warning signs or symptoms. The only way to know that you have it is from blood pressure measurements. The belief that there must be symptoms prevents many people from having regular checkups. You cannot "feel" blood pressure. You cannot tell when it's up. Very few people have any symptoms at all unless the hypertension has existed long enough for damage to occur.

> You cannot tell when your pressure is up. There's no "feeling" associated with high blood pressure. —Paul W.

> You know, just before my hypertension was diagnosed, I felt particularly well. —Debra S.

Once in a while, however, a few people may have symptoms, such as headaches, tiredness, dizziness, or nosebleeds. Most such symptoms are also common to other medical problems. They are all reasons for seeking medical help, but they may not be a sign of high blood pressure.

We will talk more about office visits, blood pressure measurements, and other tests frequently done for people with high blood pressure in Chapter 3.

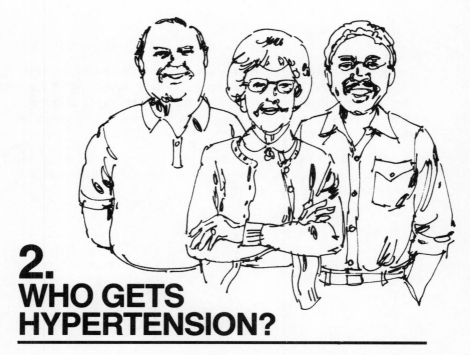

2.
WHO GETS HYPERTENSION?

Anybody can have high blood pressure. In fact, nearly 38 million Americans—more than one in five—have it. It is the most common long-term medical condition in the United States.

NO KNOWN CAUSE

Unfortunately, more than 90 percent of the time, there is no single known cause for high blood pressure. A lot of research is being done to try to find out more about it, but so far, a cause can be found in less than 10 percent of all cases. When a cause cannot be identified, the condition is called *essential hypertension*. When a cause can be identified, the condition is called *secondary hypertension*; "secondary" here means "as a result of something else."

For example, certain kidney and blood vessel diseases, hormonal disorders, and birth defects can cause high blood pressure. Some of these forms of secondary hypertension can be corrected through surgery or controlled by medication. Other causes of secondary hypertension can include certain medicines (such as birth control pills or diet pills) or even excessive amounts of licorice! In these cases, the cause can be removed, and the blood pressure should return to normal.

It is for the other 90 percent, though, that we have written this book. For you. You have what is called *essential* or *primary hypertension.* "Essential" in this sense does not mean "necessary." Rather, it is a medical term for high blood pressure that has no known cause. Since there is no cause that can be removed, *there is no cure for essential hypertension,* at least at the present time. But it can be controlled, and controlled very well. Therefore, most of the emphasis in this book is on controlling and living with essential hypertension.

PREDISPOSING RISK FACTORS

While there is usually no known cause for essential hypertension, it turns out that certain factors make some individuals more likely to develop it. *These factors do not necessarily cause high blood pressure.* But statistically, your chances of getting it are greater when one or more of the following factors apply to you:

● **Family history**. High blood pressure tends to run in families. More than half the people with high blood pressure have other family members with it. This suggests that genetic factors may play a role.

> Deep in my mind, I guess I always knew I might get high blood pressure, like my parents, so I was resigned to it.
> —Louise M.

● **Age**. People of any age can get high blood pressure, but it is more common in older age groups. It affects close to half the population above the age of 64. Hypertension is usually first diagnosed between the ages of 35 and 50. However, some evidence suggests that the tendency may be present much earlier, perhaps in the first year or two of life.

● **Sex**. Under the age of 50, high blood pressure is more common in men than in women. The rate becomes equal at about age 50, and by age 55 to 60, more women have it than men. Deaths resulting from its complications, however, occur twice as often among men.

● **Race**. For both children and adults, blacks are twice as likely to have hypertension as whites. Furthermore, blacks tend to develop it at younger ages and have higher blood pressure levels. Hypertension is the leading cause of death among blacks. For example, 100 times as many blacks die from its complications as they do from sickle cell anemia, the well-publicized genetic disease.

● **Weight**. High blood pressure is much more common in

people who are overweight than in those whose weight is normal. Close to 40 percent of all overweight people have hypertension. Weight loss tends to lower blood pressure.

• **Salt**. Salt plays a part in the body's regulation of blood pressure, but the exact relationship between salt in the diet and hypertension is not clear. Apparently, those people who have a tendency to develop high blood pressure are more likely to get it if they eat foods with a great deal of salt. Meanwhile, others who do not have this underlying tendency may be able to eat salty foods without affecting their blood pressure. Again, genetic factors may be involved.

• **Stress**. No proof has been found that directly ties stress to high blood pressure, although research into a possible relationship has been going on for some time. Some studies have reported a connection between hypertension and certain stress factors.

Thus, the environment in which people live and work may trigger high blood pressure in those who are likely to develop it in the first place. On the other hand, it is very difficult to separate environmental from genetic factors. Families usually share the same life environment, including dietary habits and often outside pressures. The fact that hypertension tends to run in families is probably due to genetic factors, but the environment may contribute. It is also not known why the rate of high blood pressure is higher among blacks. Again, it is probably a combination of lifestyle, environmental, and genetic factors.

> Being black, loving my food, and living in the 20th century sure adds up to a big risk.   —Benjamin B.

It is important to understand that these predisposing risk factors do not necessarily cause high blood pressure. And no one yet really knows why people with some or many of these factors are more likely to develop essential hypertension. At the same time, many people who have high blood pressure may not even have any of these risk factors.

> I weigh 114 pounds! People are surprised to hear that I have high blood pressure because I'm not fat.   —Louise M.

You may also have noticed that you can't "help" many of the factors. You certainly can't change your family, age, sex, or race. However, if you are overweight, eat too much salt, or are under a great deal of stress, you may be able to help control your blood pressure by making some lifestyle changes, as we show in Chapter 6.

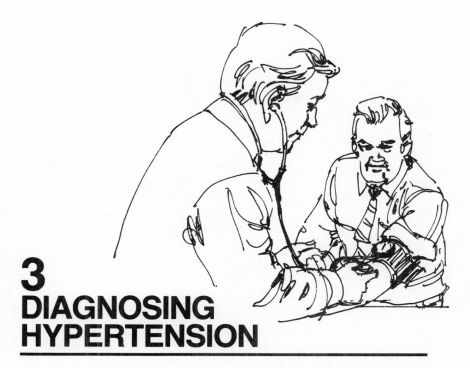

3
DIAGNOSING HYPERTENSION

As we said earlier, a specific diagnosis of hypertension is made from a series of blood pressure readings taken several days apart. In this chapter, we describe how blood pressure is measured and explain where the numbers come from. However, your doctor will be treating the whole you, and not just your blood pressure. And so, we also present the other kinds of information that your doctor will want to know.

BLOOD PRESSURE MEASUREMENTS

You've probably had your blood pressure taken dozens of times and perhaps not even thought much about how it is done or what the numbers mean. The most common device used today is called a blood pressure cuff or *sphygmomanometer* (SFIG-moe-muh-NOM-e-ter), meaning "measuring the pulse." It has several parts: a cloth or rubber cuff, which is wrapped around your arm; a rubber air bulb, which is squeezed to pump air into the cuff; and a manometer (a glass tube similar to a thermometer, which usually contains mercury, another liquid, or air) or other type of meter or clock-like gauge, which is connected to the cuff and registers the pressure reading.

The cuff is wrapped snugly around your bare upper arm just above the bend in your elbow. The doctor or nurse squeezes the bulb, pumping air into the cuff. As the cuff fills with air, the mercury in the manometer rises. Air is pumped in until the cuff presses down on the main artery, temporarily stopping the blood from flowing into your forearm.

Systolic Pressure

By placing a stethoscope on the artery just below the cuff and slowly letting the air out of the cuff, the doctor or nurse can hear the sound of blood as it begins to flow through the artery again. As the air is let out, the mercury in the tube drops, and the level of the mercury is read at the very first sound. This first sound, a thudding or tapping noise, is made by the spurt of blood pumped out by the heart with each *systole* (contraction). It begins the moment that the air pressure in the cuff is just slightly lower than the pressure in the artery.

This is your upper or *systolic pressure,* which is the tension on your artery walls that the blood produces as it is expelled from your heart. It is the maximum pressure produced by your heart and is a measure of the greatest force of the blood against the artery walls.

Diastolic Pressure

As more air is let out of the cuff, the mercury in the tube continues to drop. When the tapping sound is no longer heard through the stethoscope, the blood is flowing smoothly through the artery. A reading is taken of the mercury level when the tapping sound stops.

This reading, your lower or *diastolic pressure,* is the least amount of tension on the artery walls. This is the pressure when your heart is at rest between beats, filling up for the next contraction. It is also a measure of the constant pressure within the arterioles, the smallest arteries.

Your blood pressure reading, then, consists of two numbers. The systolic number is given first and the diastolic number second: for example, 120/80. Pressure is measured in millimeters of mercury (abbreviated as mm Hg.) The number 120 mm Hg means that your systolic pressure is equivalent to the pressure required to raise a column of mercury 120 millimeters. Don't worry if you have trouble understanding this scientific definition of blood pressure. The important point is to know your own blood pressure reading and to understand what it means to your health.

Several Readings May Be Taken

In any individual, blood pressure may differ from one arm to the other and is affected by whether you're calm or anxious, sitting or standing, at rest or following exercise. Therefore, if high blood pressure is suspected, several readings may be taken, especially at your first visit. The pressure is often read in both arms, and the arm with the higher pressure is generally used for all future measurements. Your pressure will probably also be taken while you sit, stand, and lie down. A blood pressure reading may even be taken from your leg.

THE OFFICE VISIT

Once high blood pressure has been detected, the doctor will take your medical history, perform a thorough physical examination, and order certain laboratory tests.

Your Medical History

Your *medical history* provides very useful information and involves talking honestly with your doctor, answering a series of questions, and raising any questions or concerns that you have. You will be asked whether you have previously been told that you have high blood pressure or been treated for it. The doctor will want to know if you have had any symptoms that may suggest complications of high blood pressure, such as weakness, nosebleeds, dizziness, headaches, heart palpitations, shortness of breath, and an increase in how often you need to urinate. You will be asked about any drugs that you may be taking, including birth control pills, hormones, and cold remedies. Other questions will concern possible symptoms associated with kidney, heart, or blood vessel disease, all of which can be complications of untreated hypertension.

The doctor will need a complete picture of your health over your lifetime, as well as information on the health of your family members. In particular, you will be asked whether you or anyone in your family has had diabetes, a kidney disease, a stroke, or other cardiovascular disease. Your family's history is especially important because high blood pressure is frequently hereditary.

The doctor also needs to know about your current lifestyle, to find out about other factors that put you at risk for high blood pressure or cardiovascular disease. Thus, you will be asked about your job, your relations with your family members, your habits, and your overall impression of how things are going.

The Physical Exam

You will have a complete *physical examination,* which includes checking your weight and taking samples of blood and urine for various laboratory tests, described below. The examination will indicate the overall state of your health.

The doctor will want to find out whether hypertension has caused any damage to your heart, blood vessels, eyes, or kidneys. Your eyes provide one of the earliest clues. Using an *ophthalmoscope,* the doctor can see the tiny blood vessels in the retina, at the back of the eye. These are the only blood vessels that can be seen from the outside; they may be representative of the condition of all the arterioles throughout your body.

Your heart sounds will be checked with a stethoscope. Changes in sound may indicate the effect of high blood pressure on the pumping action of your heart muscle. With high blood pressure, the heart may become enlarged. This enlargement can sometimes be detected by tapping the chest and listening to the sounds. The doctor will also listen with a stethoscope for signs of fluid in your lungs.

Finally, your pulse will be taken in several places, to check for signs of reduced blood flow resulting from narrowed arteries. And your neck, lungs, abdomen, kidneys, and arms and legs will be checked for swellings, reflexes, or other signs of a problem.

LABORATORY TESTS

Because there is no known specific cause for 90 percent of all cases of hypertension, extensive laboratory tests are seldom necessary. Certain tests, however, are usually done as part of the routine workup.

Blood and Urine Tests

One of the most important tests is a *urinalysis,* a detailed study of the urine. The levels of protein, blood, and glucose (sugar) in the urine are carefully measured to see whether your high blood pressure may be due to an underlying problem such as a kidney disorder.

Blood samples will be checked for the presence of anemia, the level of proteins, and the amount of potassium and sodium. In addition, tests for cholesterol and other blood fats may be done.

If any of these tests suggests that your high blood pressure may have been caused by a disorder of the kidneys or adrenal glands, or that potential heart problems may exist, further tests would be recommended.

Electrocardiogram

This test, called an EKG or ECG, is commonly done to see whether your heart has been affected by high blood pressure. It is usually done in the doctor's office and takes only a few minutes. Small disks called *leads* are placed on your chest, wrists, and ankles and connected by wires to a recording machine. As your heart beats, the leads pick up signals of your heart's activity. The signals are transmitted to a pen, which traces your heart's electrical activity, rate and rhythm onto a strip of moving graph paper in the EKG machine.

Each contraction of a normal heartbeat is shown by a specific and regular wave pattern on the paper. EKG patterns may reveal disturbances in the blood supply to the heart muscle or irregularities in the heartbeat.

Other Tests

Chest x-rays can provide information about the size of your heart and are especially helpful for comparing changes in heart size over the years. For that reason, or if the doctor suspects that your heart is already enlarged, a chest x-ray may be recommended.

Echocardiography is another laboratory procedure that can be helpful in deciding if the heart is enlarged. This test uses *ultrasound,* or high-frequency sound waves, to get an image of the heart. Like sonar, which measures the depths of things at sea, echo-cardiography sends sound waves to different spots around the heart. The sound waves come back as echoes, which are recorded and plotted. The resulting *echocardiogram* is shown on a screen or computer.

Some or all of these tests will be done during the initial diagnosis of high blood pressure. Later, your doctor may repeat them to measure your progress during treatment.

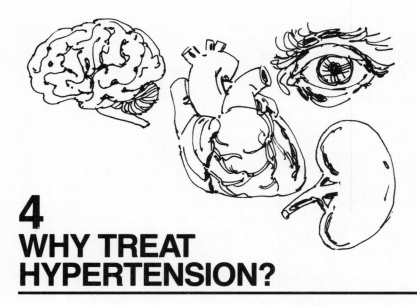

4 WHY TREAT HYPERTENSION?

Since you probably feel fine and aren't really "sick," you may wonder why you should lower your blood pressure. The main reason for treating high blood pressure is to *prevent* its consequences. If it is not treated, blood pressure will often go higher. Eventually, it can affect your whole circulatory or *cardiovascular system*—that is, your heart and all your blood vessels—and therefore every organ in your body. Untreated hypertension can be present for 15 to 20 years before symptoms occur. And, most importantly, symptoms often don't usually appear until some permanent damage to body organs has been done.

> People with high blood pressure aren't sick—high blood pressure is a *condition*. There are many things that can be done to keep them from getting sick, though.   —Dr. M.

Thus, even though hypertension is not a disease, its presence increases your risk of developing certain conditions. Life insurance companies, for example, place a great deal of emphasis on it. According to their calculations, even a small increase in blood pressure is believed to shorten life expectancy. The most serious effects are heart attacks, heart failure, strokes, kidney failure, and blood vessel damage in other organs such as the eyes or legs. People with high blood pressure are three to seven times more likely to develop one of these conditions than are people whose blood pressure is normal. Economically, hypertension and its consequences amount to an estimated $8 billion a year in medical costs, lost work productivity, and lost wages.

> I had no idea that I had high blood pressure until one day, while sewing, I went completely blind in one eye, from a hemorrhage. I was hospitalized immediately. —Debra S.

Fortunately, the serious consequences of high blood pressure can usually be prevented when hypertension is diagnosed, treated, and controlled. By treating and controlling your blood pressure now, you can help prevent serious complications and increase your life expectancy.

In the rest of this chapter, we describe how *untreated* hypertension can affect the body. Our purpose is not to scare you, but rather to help you understand why it is so important to treat your high blood pressure regardless of how well you feel. There really are things that you can do that will make a difference.

> For a while, I didn't take my high blood pressure very seriously and sometimes didn't bother to take my medicines. Now I know that I have to take them regularly. —Benjamin B.

RISK FACTORS FOR CARDIOVASCULAR DISEASE

One of the most serious aspects of untreated hypertension is its connection with *cardiovascular disease*. This term refers to any disease of the heart or blood vessels; strokes and heart attacks are the most common. High blood pressure is thought to be the major *risk factor* associated with cardiovascular disease. In Chapter 2, we talked about how certain factors in your background may have made you more likely to get hypertension. Similarly, factors in your lifestyle and background increase your chances of developing cardiovascular disease.

Some risk factors you can't "help" and therefore can't change. Doctors call these *unmodifiable risk factors*. In particular, you are more likely to develop coronary artery disease if:

- You have close blood relatives who have had it. Your risk is greater if someone in your family had a heart attack under the age of 50.
- You are male.
- You have diabetes. (Diabetes, of course, can be controlled medically, but its presence is still a risk factor.)
- You are over 40.

Since you can't do much about those factors, we'd rather talk about the ones that you may be able to do something about. *Modifiable risk factors* are those over which you have some control. They often result from the way you live—the things you eat and the things you do. According to the American Heart Association, the major modifiable risk factors that would make you more likely to develop cardiovascular disease are:

- high blood pressure.
- cigarette smoking.
- a high level of cholesterol in your blood.
- overweight.
- a lot of stress and tension in your life.

In addition, other habits may influence these risk factors. For example, if you don't get enough exercise you may gain weight.

While the experts don't know exactly how these risk factors *cause* heart attacks and strokes, there is a strong relationship between them and cardiovascular disease. Of course, not everyone with some of or even all these risk factors will develop a serious problem, and some people with cardiovascular disease do not have any of them. But *your risks* are much greater if some of them apply to you. And the more that you have, the higher your risks are. *Combining risk factors is not like adding them—it's more like multiplying them.*

In the following pages, we discuss cardiovascular disease and then talk about how these factors may put you at risk. You may have noticed that several of them are the same as the predisposing risk factors for hypertension, discussed in Chapter 2. It should be clear, then, that by controlling your risk factors for hypertension you improve your situation against cardiovascular disease. In Chapter 6, we talk more about the particular risk factors that apply to both high blood pressure and cardiovascular disease. By lowering your blood pressure and reducing your other risks, you can really do a lot for yourself.

> I know it isn't a sure thing, but I believe that as long as I remember to take medicine for my high blood pressure, I can help fight off strokes and heart attacks.   —Louise M.

ATHEROSCLEROSIS AND CARDIOVASCULAR DISEASE

The inside walls of blood vessels are normally smooth and flexible, letting the blood flow through them easily. Over the years, however, fats and other materials carried in the bloodstream begin to cling to the walls. As these deposits or *plaques* build up, the space inside the vessels (called the *lumen*) may become narrowed or blocked, restricting the flow of blood. Narrowed arteries have a harder time delivering enough blood and oxygen to various cells and organs. Without proper nourishment, cells may die and organs may begin to fail.

The process of plaque buildup is called *atherosclerosis*, or *hardening of the arteries*. It is similar to what happens when rust collects inside old iron pipes; the flow of water begins to slow down, eventually can only drip through, and may even stop.

Atherosclerosis is a slow, progressive disease that may begin as early as childhood. It often takes years for the plaques to build up enough to slow down the blood flow. It can happen inside any artery in the body and can lead to many types of circulatory problems. Two of the major problems due to atherosclerosis are heart attacks and strokes.

Coronary Artery Disease

Atherosclerosis is especially likely to present a problem when it develops in the *coronary arteries*. These are the small blood vessels that carry blood deep into the heart muscle. If plaques build up inside these arteries and blood can't get to the heart, the heart muscle may become "starved" for oxygen. When atherosclerosis involves one or more of the coronary arteries, it is called *coronary artery disease*.

Coronary artery disease is by far the leading cause of serious heart problems, including *angina pectoris* (meaning "pain in the chest") and *myocardial infarction* (a type of heart attack). Angina pectoris, or angina, occurs when the heart *temporarily* does not get enough oxygen. The signal is a discomfort or pain, usually in the chest, and it is generally brief. A myocardial infarction can occur when the heart muscle gets *very little* or *no* oxygen for a period of time. The area of heart muscle that loses its oxygen supply is permanently damaged and the heart muscle cells in that area die.

Strokes

If atherosclerosis develops in an artery that leads to the brain, the result may be a stroke. When a blood vessel to the brain is blocked, the nerve cells in that area of the brain are deprived of oxygen and can no longer function. The part of the body that those cells control can no longer function, either. The narrowing or blockage may be caused by atherosclerosis alone. It also may be caused by a blood clot (*thrombus*) that forms around a plaque in an artery wall (cerebral thrombosis) or by a blood clot or other material that has been carried by the bloodstream from another part of the vascular system (cerebral embolism).

Another type of stroke can occur if a blood vessel leading to the brain ruptures or hemorrhages. Called an *intracranial hemorrhage* (meaning "bleeding within the skull"), this can occur because a blood vessel is defective or weakened from disease.

Other Blood Vessel Problems

Atherosclerosis can cause narrowing in the blood vessels anywhere in the body. It can eventually affect any part of the circulatory system. For example, some people develop circulatory problems in their legs and feet due to narrowed blood vessels. Other parts of the body that may be affected are the kidneys and the eyes.

HIGH BLOOD PRESSURE AS A RISK FACTOR

Hypertension is one of the most important risk factors leading to cardiovascular disease. It may not actually *cause* cardiovascular disease, but it does play a large role in the development of atherosclerosis. It also affects your heart in other ways. However, as you will see in later chapters, there is a lot that you can do to keep high blood pressure from being so damaging.

> Most of my patients are aware of the complications of untreated high blood pressure. In fact, many of them think it's even worse than it is. I don't want to scare them. I have to stress that these are "maybe's."   —Dr. W.

High Blood Pressure and Narrowed Arteries

Atherosclerosis may develop from a number of factors. High blood pressure, however, seems to speed up the process of fat buildup in blood vessel walls. As blood flows through your body, it puts pressure on the inside walls of the arteries, which stretch and contract as the blood pulses through. When blood pressure is consistently high, it pushes against the artery walls with extra force. Gradually, the muscular layer of the artery walls becomes hard and thick. This causes the arteries to lose their elasticity, and the space inside the blood vessels becomes smaller. If your arteries are already diseased by atherosclerosis, high blood pressure worsens this process. Thus, we have a continuing cycle: Atherosclerosis makes the vessel openings smaller; the narrowed vessels make the blood pressure rise; and more fat is deposited on the vessel walls.

Over time, narrowed arteries can lead to a number of serious complications, including heart attacks and strokes. People with high blood pressure are five times more likely to have a heart attack than are people whose blood pressure is normal, and 90 percent of all stroke victims have high blood pressure.

Harder Work for Your Heart

When blood pressure is high, your heart must pump harder to keep the blood moving. Like the muscles in your legs, which get bigger the more you exercise, the heart may likewise become bigger. In this case, unlike the legs, bigger does not necessarily mean stronger. Eventually the heart muscle loses some of its pumping power.

At some point, the heart may no longer be strong enough to keep the blood circulating. It may gradually begin to fail. The flow of blood throughout the body slows down. The result is congestion, or a backup of fluid, in the circulatory system. This condition is called *congestive heart failure*. "Failure," here, means that the heart just doesn't work as well as it should. High blood pressure is one of the most common causes of congestive heart failure.

CIGARETTE SMOKING AND YOUR HEART

The damaging effects of cigarette smoking on the lungs are well-known. But smoking is also damaging to the heart and blood vessels. In particular, coronary artery disease is more common and more severe among smokers than among nonsmokers. Cigarette smokers are two to three times more likely to have a heart attack than are nonsmokers. And following a heart attack, cigarette smokers have a poorer chance of recovery.

Cigarette smoking alters the normal circulatory system by:
● Stimulating the heart, making it beat faster, and narrowing the blood vessels.
● Causing carbon monoxide to be absorbed into the blood in the lungs, replacing oxygen. This decreases the supply of oxygen that gets to the heart and body tissues.

• Making the blood more likely to clot and less able to dissolve clots.

• Causing "extra" or irregular heartbeats.

The encouraging news is that as soon as you stop smoking, your body will benefit. You probably can't undo the damage that has been done to the arteries. But as soon as you put out your last cigarette, your heart and lungs begin to function better.

Many smokers, however, believe that because damage has been done, it's too late to quit. *It's never too late to quit!* The risk of a heart attack starts dropping once you haven't smoked for 1 year. And, after 15 years without smoking, your risk becomes almost the same as that for anyone else your age who has never smoked. The risk of death from other causes also decreases. Regardless of your age, quitting can improve your overall health and your life expectancy.

CHOLESTEROL AND OTHER FATS

Several kinds of fatty materials are carried in the bloodstream. These fats are called *lipids*, one of which is *cholesterol*. Cholesterol is made by the body, mostly by the liver, and is found in many foods. Egg yolks, organ meats such as liver and kidneys, and certain kinds of shellfish are high in cholesterol. Although the body needs a certain amount of this waxy, fatty substance, too much of it is not good. As they flow through the bloodstream, cholesterol and other lipids can stick to the artery walls. A high level of cholesterol in the blood is one of the chief causes of atherosclerosis.

In general, the higher the blood cholesterol level the more likely you are to develop cardiovascular disease. Fortunately, cholesterol levels can usually be lowered sufficiently by making changes in your diet.

In addition, scientists have discovered that it may be the kind of cholesterol in the blood, as well as the amount, that is important. Most cholesterol is carried in the bloodstream in combination with protein. This is called *lipoprotein*. The two main types of lipoproteins are—a "good" type called *HDL* (for *high-density lipoprotein*) and a "bad" type called *LDL* (for *low-density lipoprotein*). The higher the ratio of HDL cholesterol to total cholesterol, the lower the risk of heart attack.

Your doctor can test for both the amount and type of cholesterol in your blood and will work with you to lower total cholesterol and raise the level of HDL cholesterol. In addition, if you have high cholesterol *and* if you have children, it may be a good idea to have their cholesterol levels checked and to start watching their diets, too. High blood pressure, high cholesterol levels, and cardiovascular disease all tend to run in families.

> I'm 39, and have just begun to work to lower my cholesterol. But my son's only 8.... The earlier he starts watching the fats in his diet, the better his chances are.   —Dr. N.

Different Kinds of Fats

In addition to foods that contain cholesterol, other kinds of fats from food can affect the level of cholesterol in the blood. All fats are a form of food energy, and some fat is essential to a healthy diet. But almost 40 percent of the average American diet consists of fats, which is probably much more than we need. Some of these fats turn into cholesterol in the blood. Furthermore, fats have more than twice as many calories, ounce for ounce, as protein and carbohydrates do. Therefore, many doctors recommend that people control the *amount* and *kind* of fat in their diet. *The amount of fat you eat affects your weight; the kind of fat you eat affects your cholesterol level.*

Most fats are made up of different types of substances. Two kinds are *saturated fats* and *unsaturated fats*. Some saturated fat turns into cholesterol in the body, while unsaturated fats may help lower blood cholesterol. Saturated fats usually come from animal and dairy products, such as meats, cream, cheese, and butter; they are generally solid at room temperature. Unsaturated fats, which come from vegetable products, are usually liquid at room temperature; corn oil, soybean oil, and other vegetable oils are examples. Note, however, that a few liquid fats (such as coconut oil and palm oil) are saturated rather than unsaturated.

Therefore, it may be recommended that you reduce the amount of saturated fats in your diet. It may also be helpful to *replace* saturated with unsaturated fats whenever possible. For example, use certain types of margarine instead of butter. The calories and amount of fat are the same in both kinds, but the unsaturated fat may be less harmful. (See Appendix I, no. 1, p. 67 for other sources of information on dietary fats.)

EXCESS WEIGHT

If you weigh too much, an additional work load is placed on your heart. For every pound of fat on your body, your heart has to pump blood through an extra three-quarters of a mile of blood vessels. And it does this about 70 times a minute. Even when resting, an overweight body works harder to breathe and needs more oxygen.

No one knows for sure whether being overweight causes cardiovascular disease, but there is at least an association between excess weight and increased risk. For example, the heart attack rate for people who are 30 pounds overweight is twice that for people of normal weight. On average, an extra 30 pounds may decrease your life expectancy by 4 years. And the risk goes up as your weight goes up. If you do have a heart attack, furthermore, your chances for a good recovery are better if your weight is normal.

Being overweight is also linked with other problems. Over-weight people are three times as likely to have high blood pressure and four times as likely to have diabetes. They often have high levels of cholesterol and other fats in their blood as well. And, of course, all these things compound the risks for heart disease.

Weight loss has many benefits. It is often accompanied by a drop in blood pressure, as we discuss in Chapter 6. It may help lower cholesterol levels, and it is frequently helpful in controlling diabetes. By easing the strain on your heart, a weight loss will give you more energy. Thus, you will tire less easily and can exercise more, which will improve your cardiovascular fitness.

STRESS

All of us have stress in our lives—bills to pay, children to raise, tension on the job. Stress can result from outside events such as driving in traffic or business pressures, interpersonal relationships such as family tension or arguments, and internal causes such as worry or depression. Even happy events—a wedding, a new home, an exciting football game—can cause stress. Indeed, some stress helps make life interesting.

During periods of stress, your body reacts in a number of ways, such as:
● You breathe more rapidly and deeply, taking in more oxygen.
● Your red blood cells flow faster through your bloodstream, carrying more oxygen to your heart and muscles.
● Your heart beats faster and your blood pressure rises, so that your heart and muscles get extra nutrients and oxygen faster.

• Your blood supply is rerouted from areas where it is not needed at the moment—such as the surface of your skin or your digestive system—to your muscles and brain, where it is needed.

• Your blood's ability to clot increases, so that if an injury occurs, less blood is lost from the wound.

Usually, your body reacts to stress when necessary and then returns to "normal." You probably aren't even aware of your body's responses in many cases. You may not even know that you are under stress.

The experts don't really know what role stress plays in cardiovascular disease. Some say that stress by itself may not be related at all, while others say that people who are always under stress have a much higher risk. And still others believe that it is not the stress itself but how you *react* to it and cope with it that may be the key. In other words, your personality may matter. People who are aggressive, competitive, and hard-driving are more likely to react to stressful events with that same kind of intensity. They are also somewhat more likely to develop cardiovascular disease. Easygoing, relaxed, and patient people, on the other hand, seem to handle stress more easily.

EXERCISE

According to some studies, people who get little or no exercise on the job or through their activities may be more likely to have a heart attack. And people who are physically fit recover faster from heart attacks than do people who are not. On the other hand, nobody really knows whether physical activity itself can help prevent heart attacks and strokes.

While a direct relationship between exercise and cardiovascular disease has not been proved, regular exercise does do good things to your heart and body:

• Your lungs can take up oxygen better, and your heart pumps blood more efficiently. In a physically fit person, the heart beats more slowly but more forcefully.

• Your circulation is improved, making your lungs, heart, and other muscles work together better.

• Exercise may lower your LDL cholesterol level and raise the HDL portion, thus slowing down the buildup of plaques.

• Exercise gives you more physical strength and improves your muscle tone. Thus, you can do more and will tire less easily.

• Exercise may improve your mental state. You may be able to handle stress and tension better, relax more easily, and sleep better. A well-exercised body generally "feels" better.

• Along with a proper diet, it can help control your weight.

Exercise as a form of treatment for cardiovascular disease is a fairly recent development. More studies need to be done, but some early findings suggest that with proper exercise training, some people may be able to reduce the total demand on their hearts by slowing the heart rate and increasing its pumping capacity. The heart's efficiency is improved, so it can do the same amount of work with less effort. There is also some evidence that regular and frequent exercise may reduce blood pressure.

> Exercise helps make the heart more efficient. Like a more efficient car, you can get more miles to the gallon, so to speak. Even if your heart should have a problem, you can go farther on it. —Dr. C.

A good exercise program may help improve the heart's blood supply. Some experts think that a significant amount of exercise may increase the size of the arteries, letting more blood reach the heart muscle. It is also possible, but not yet proved, that exercise may lead to the development of *collateral circulation*. Collateral (meaning "substitute" or "side by side") circulation occurs when small vessels from branches of the coronary arteries join up with others, grow tiny new vessels, and form a detour for blood to flow around a blocked or narrowed artery. Collateral circulation can sometimes help compensate for blocked arteries. If collateral circulation has developed and a heart attack occurs, the attack may be less severe. Also, the chances of avoiding a second heart attack seem to be better.

SUMMARY

As we have shown, high blood pressure can be serious. In particular, it is thought to be the most important risk factor for cardiovascular disease. And when linked with several other risk factors, most importantly high cholesterol and cigarette smoking, it can present a very substantial risk.

On the other hand, two points are in your favor. First, now you know that you have high blood pressure. Treatment today is highly successful, and blood pressure can almost always be controlled. By controlling it, you will decrease your risks of cardiovascular disease. Second, you can help yourself even more by thinking about your other risk factors at the same time. Identifying risk factors and working to change them are two of the major steps we can all take to increase our chances of a longer, more healthy life.

An encouraging note is that the death rate from cardiovascular disease has been declining steadily for the past twenty years or so. The rate has dropped by more than 20 percent, and the number of strokes has declined by even more, perhaps by 30 to 40 percent. The exact reasons for these decreases are not certain, but most experts agree that some of the change has occurred because so many Americans are controlling their risk factors. And one of the risk factors that is being controlled better than ever is high blood pressure.

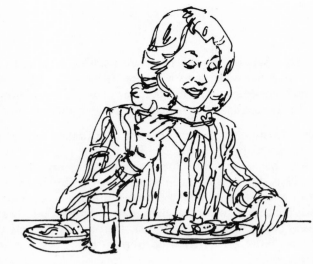

5
TREATMENT APPROACHES

Knowledge about hypertension and forms of treatment is really quite new. Experts have been aware of atherosclerosis for some time. Many of them believed that high blood pressure somehow acted to compensate for hardened arteries. Their theory was that blood pressure increased in order to push blood through the arteries. But it is now known that the increased pressure weakens the already damaged arteries.

When doctors first began to understand the damaging effects of high blood pressure, there wasn't much that they could do to treat it. Then drugs were developed that were able to lower pressure in some people, but they frequently caused bad reactions. The treatment was sometimes worse than the condition. Also, several different drugs were often required, with complicated schedules for taking them. Therefore, most doctors treated only those people with very high blood pressure.

For the same reasons, many people never followed through on their treatment or stopped taking the drugs once their pressure was lowered. Doctors, not fully realizing the problems of treatment, didn't always follow up to see that the blood pressure stayed under control.

WHO SHOULD BE TREATED?

We are more fortunate today. The drugs available now are much more successful in lowering blood pressure. The side effects are fewer, and the schedules for taking the drugs are easier to follow.

At the same time, recent research has shown two important things. First, as we mentioned in the last chapter, death rates from heart attacks and strokes have dropped considerably in the last several years. Moreover, many more people with high blood pressure are being detected and treated than ever before. These two facts are probably related. Treating—rather than ignoring—hypertension clearly pays off.

Second, research has also shown that people with mild hypertension benefit from treatment, too. In the past, doctors thought that "slightly high" blood pressure was probably not harmful. They used to keep an eye on those people to make sure that the pressure didn't go too high, but they seldom prescribed treatment. According to recent studies, however, people with mild hypertension who are treated are less likely to have a stroke than those who are not treated. There may also be a reduction in the frequency of heart disease.

> My hypertension is mild, and I feel fine. Also, my friends seemed to downplay my condition. Therefore, I began to get a little careless about my drugs and diet. I guess I didn't realize how important it is to treat mild hypertension.
> —Nancy L.

So, today, many medical experts believe that *everyone with an average diastolic pressure of 90 mm Hg or above should begin working with a doctor to get it lowered.*

KINDS OF TREATMENT

Essential hypertension can be controlled, not cured. Treatment thus aims first to lower your diastolic blood pressure to below a predetermined goal, if possible, and then to keep it down. Most physicians agree that below 90 mm Hg is an acceptable goal, though many aim for a lower figure if possible.

> Although "89" may be a goal, I like to try to get blood pressure even lower. The lower, the better.   —Dr. M.

Drugs have usually been the main form of treatment, and drug therapy today is very successful. Most people will need to take only one or two drugs. Some people, however, may require several. In some cases, blood pressure can be lowered by other means, such as by dieting, cutting down on salt, exercising or learning to relax. All these various forms of treatment are discussed in the next two chapters.

Actually, to some extent, it doesn't matter *how* you lower your blood pressure, as long as you do it. Therefore, you and your doctor will try to find the program that works best for you. It will probably involve a combination of drugs and minor lifestyle changes.

Many people, when they first learn that they have high blood pressure, are afraid that they'll have to rearrange their entire lives. This false belief, sadly, causes some people to stop right there and never follow through on their therapy. The fact is that very few people with hypertension have to make major changes in their lives. The changes that may be recommended are usually small, and they get easier as time goes on.

> It's unfortunate to have this condition, but if you take the drugs to keep your blood pressure lowered, I've found that nothing in your life really changes. —Paul W.

Your particular program will depend on who you are, what you want to do and can do, how high your blood pressure is, and other things about you and your health, such as your age, sex, and the presence of other risk factors for cardiovascular diseases. *Your program will be individualized*—that is, tailored specifically for you as an individual. It will not be the same as someone else's.

Because there is no real cure for essential hypertension, bringing your pressure down is only the first step. After that, you need to keep it down, or it will just go right back up. This is why we talk about *controlling* high blood pressure.

Since you are beginning a long-term project, it is important that your treatment program be something you are comfortable with. Treatment is not considered successful if it interferes significantly with your normal life. It may take some time before you and your doctor find a plan that is comfortable for you. But it's worth the effort. For everybody, there's some combination of treatment that is best.

> I have changed my eating and drinking habits. I have a darling foster child and a wife I love, and I want to stay well and live a long time. —Benjamin B.

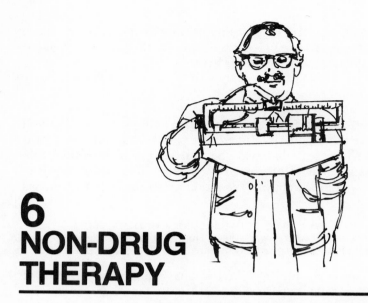

6
NON-DRUG
THERAPY

Blood pressure can be lowered in a number of ways. In Chapter 2, we mentioned that being overweight, eating a lot of salt, and having a good deal of stress in your life may have made you more likely to develop high blood pressure. The reverse is that you *may* be able to lower your blood pressure by losing weight, cutting down on salt, and learning to relieve your stress. If your pressure is only slightly high, such lifestyle changes may be enough to bring it within the normal range; you may not need any drugs. For others, these changes may result in fewer drugs or lower dosages. If your blood pressure is not adequately controlled after reasonable efforts with lifestyle changes, then there should be no hesitation in proceeding directly to drug therapy.

LOSING WEIGHT

Being overweight does not necessarily cause high blood pressure, but there is a strong relationship between the two. For example, overweight people are three times as likely to have hypertension as are people of normal weight. Even a gradual weight gain over the years, especially during early adulthood, is linked with high blood pressure.

We pointed out the close association between excess weight and cardiovascular disease in Chapter 4. High blood pressure makes the association even stronger. With high blood pressure, your heart is already working hard against the pressure in your arteries. Extra body weight—even a few pounds—increases the volume of blood and puts a greater burden on your heart.

The Benefits of Losing Weight

If you are overweight, your doctor will probably urge you to lose those extra pounds. But even if your weight is normal, it is important to keep it that way. Several studies have shown that weight loss is often accompanied by a decrease in blood pressure. And if the weight is kept off, the blood pressure generally remains lower.

> If I could do it over again, I would try very hard not to put on extra weight when I was young. I'm having a *terrible* time trying to take it off now that I'm older.   —Debra S.

For some people, weight loss may be the only treatment required. For mild hypertension, it is sometimes the first step. Drugs and other therapy may not be started until your doctor sees how well you do with weight loss first. And for many other people, losing weight may mean fewer drugs or lower dosages.

The key, however, is to keep the weight off. This is often the hardest part. If you regain the weight, which often happens, your blood pressure will just go up again. So, many doctors are reluctant to put too much emphasis on weight loss as the only form of therapy.

Controlling Your Diet

Even when the amount and kinds of food eaten stay the same, people usually gain weight after age 25 unless they do something about it. In general, the body needs 10 fewer calories a day for each year of age older than 25. One hundred extra calories a day (about 10 potato chips) adds up to about 10 pounds a year. It's easy to see how people put on weight over the years.

To lose or control your weight, you need to think in terms of supply and demand. If you supply your body with more food (calories) than it needs, and if you don't burn off those calories by exercise and everyday activities, you will gain weight. Your body's oversupply of calories will be deposited as fat. The aim of a diet, then, is to use up the stored fat. For this, you will need to cut down on calories (the supply) or increase your activities (the demand), or both.

Help for Dieting

There is no sure or easy way to lose weight, and even keeping it under control is a lifelong job. If you are overweight, it is most likely to be due to poor eating habits. You can't get rid of these old habits overnight, but you can develop new ones that will help you consume less and eat food that is better for you.

Most people try to diet on their own. If you are seriously overweight or need to control both the types and the amounts of food you eat, you may want help. Dieting is seldom easy, and you may want advice from doctors, dietitians, or nurses because:

- They can help you plan a diet that still makes eating pleasurable.
- They can help you change your eating habits.
- They can advise you on setting *realistic* goals regarding how much and how fast you should expect to lose.
- They can help you understand why fad diets, crash diets, and some reducing aids seldom work.

In addition to professional assistance, many excellent self-help groups and publications are available to aid people in planning and following a weight-loss program (see Appendix I, no. 2, p. 67). You don't have to be a super cook, and diets don't have to be dull and tiresome.

If you do need to control your weight, don't be discouraged if your good intentions go out the window once in a while.

CUTTING DOWN ON SALT

Sodium is one of several minerals required by the body. It occurs naturally in almost all food, but you probably know it best in the form of table salt, which is 40 percent sodium and 60 percent chloride.

Salt and High Blood Pressure

The relationship between salt and high blood pressure is not completely understood, although some studies have shown a link. Too much sodium causes the body to retain water. When water is not eliminated, the volume of blood in circulation is increased. This, in turn, increases the pressure in the arteries.

Therefore, it is thought that too much salt in the diet may contribute to hypertension, especially in people who have an underlying tendency to develop high blood pressure. Other people can eat salt with little or no effect on their blood pressure.

However, most experts agree that the American diet is heavy on salt. Most of us consume about 10 grams (or 2 teaspoons) of salt a day. The amount our bodies actually need is found naturally in foods. We do not need the extra salt that we add in cooking or at the table. The U.S. dietary guidelines recommend that all of us restrict our salt consumption to less than 5 grams (about 1 teaspoon) a day. This figure represents all sources of sodium, including naturally occurring sodium and that hidden in processed foods.

Some Restriction Is Often Recommended

Treatment for hypertension often includes at least some restriction of salt. Severe restriction—to less than one-half a gram a day—is seldom necessary and usually not practical. Although such a strict diet will reduce blood pressure even in people with severe or malignant hypertension, it is extremely hard to stick to, and the problem of water retention can usually be solved in another way. In fact, this is a good example of how treatment for high blood pressure has improved in recent years. Not too long ago, people were put on very strict salt-free diets (such as rice and fruit only!) to lower blood pressure. Today, diuretics help wash the excess salt out of the body, so such diets are not necessary.

It is more common to aim for a moderate restriction of salt, to about 1 teaspoon per day. In some cases, reducing salt intake to this level may lower blood pressure as much as 10 mm Hg. Sometimes it may be the only treatment necessary. Or it may mean fewer drugs or lower dosages.

A reduced-salt diet does not have to be bland and tasteless. The desire for salt may be an acquired taste—that is, it is something you learn to like and then continue to want. It may also be "unlearned," although it may be hard at first. You may have to give up some of your favorite foods, but there is a lot left to choose from. In fact, many people later claim that their food begins to taste better without salt.

> I use only a little salt in cooking but none at the table. Now that I'm used to it, the submarine sandwiches I sometimes buy for lunch taste too salty. But I love ham; I can't give that up. —Benjamin B.

Simple Guidelines

Reducing your salt to a teaspoon or less a day is fairly easily done by following these guidelines:

- Buy fresh meats, vegetables, and fruits.
- Add little or no salt in preparing foods. Try herbs or lemon juice instead.
- Add little or no salt to your food at the table.
- Avoid canned, processed, or convenience foods, such as TV dinners. Read the labels carefully on all processed and packaged foods before choosing. Note that not all dietetic food is salt free. In fact, some low-calorie foods have a lot of salt. Moreover, with only a moderate reduction in salt, dietetic foods should not be necessary.
- Avoid obviously salty foods such as bacon, sausages, pretzels, some cheeses, pickles, and mustard.

> I was told not to use salt, and usually I don't. But I've got to have salt on mashed potatoes! —Debra S.

In addition to obviously salty snacks, foods that are high in sodium include most frozen or prepared foods, canned vegetables and soups, soft drinks, bottled salad dressings, luncheon meats, baking soda, baking powder, and monosodium glutamate (MSG, often used as Accént). Other foods with a lot of sodium may be surprising: Some cereals and puddings, for example, have twice as much sodium per serving as do peanuts and potato chips! And even cottage cheese has more sodium than peanuts have.

The charts in Appendix II, p. 69, compare a typical day's meals, one high in sodium and one low. Also listed are several common foods, comparing a high-sodium version (for example, canned) with a low-sodium version (for example, fresh). These lists, of course, are not complete. Rather, they are included to show you the wide range of sodium content and the kinds of trade-offs you can make.

> Advice? Trust your doctor and give your salt shaker to your worst enemy. —Benjamin B.

If your dietary changes are more complicated, requiring salt restriction and less saturated fat and cholesterol, you may need help in planning meals. A dietitian can help you draw up lists of good and bad foods and teach you how to make your diet nutritionally balanced as well as tasty. That's the key: If the food doesn't taste good, you'll have a hard time sticking with any diet. A number of low-salt cookbooks and other publications give advice on seasonings and ways to alter recipes. (See Appendix I, no. 4, p. 67.)

RELIEVING STRESS

The experts don't really know how stress relates to hypertension. One of the body's responses to stress is a temporary increase in blood pressure. But the pressure usually returns to "normal" after the stressful situation is over. Contrary to popular belief, there is no proof directly linking stress with sustained high blood pressure. Some studies, though, suggest that people who are always under stress have a higher risk. On the other hand, the connection may be like that between stress and cardiovascular disease: Many researchers believe that it is not the stress itself but how you react to it and cope with it that may be a factor.

In any case, some people with high blood pressure may benefit by learning to relieve stress. Sometimes, the benefit may be direct—a drop in blood pressure may result. At other times, the benefit may be indirect—you may simply feel better.

While you can't avoid stress completely, you can try to master it. You can try to become aware of stressful situations, avoid some of them, and learn how to cope better with the unavoidable. Some things, of course, can't be controlled. Decide when to give in and when to fight back, saving your reserves for when it really matters. Both overreacting and not reacting can bring on more stress.

Relaxation Techniques

In recent years, there has been a lot of interest in using various methods of relaxation as a means of lowering or controlling blood pressure. Some of the more popular methods are yoga, transcendental meditation, biofeedback, and the relaxation response. The proponents of the techniques claim that people who practice them regularly can successfully gain control over certain bodily functions that are normally regulated by the central nervous system, such as heartbeat, body temperature, and blood pressure.

Some modest success has been reported in lowering blood pressure by relaxation methods. For some people, at least for short periods of time, any of the techniques may work. They all require training and daily practice, although the relaxation response can be self-taught. Relaxation methods are seldom a substitute for drugs, diet, or other therapy. And they don't appeal to everyone. Furthermore, some of them may be expensive.

More research needs to be done on the possible benefits of the various methods. The biggest question at this point is whether the effects last after the individual stops practicing regularly.

Exercise

An exercise program may be beneficial for people with hypertension. Although there is no proof yet, some studies have suggested that regular and frequent exercise may reduce blood pressure.

Exercise has other benefits, too. (See Appendix I, no. 5, p. 67.) Along with a proper diet, it can help with weight loss and then keep your weight under control. It raises your HDL or "good" cholesterol levels, as well. Exercise, of course, can increase your physical strength. Thus, you can do more and will tire less easily. Some people simply feel better and more relaxed after exercising. It may be a good way to relieve tension and stress.

> I take walks occasionally, but I do it more as a form of relaxation than for the sake of exercising. —Debra S.

Before beginning an exercise program, however, discuss it with your doctor. The wrong exercise for your condition can be harmful.

The best exercise is rhythmic and repetitive and uses your large muscles, such as your back and lower legs. Aerobic exercise of this type makes your whole cardiovascular system work. It includes such activities as walking, jogging, cycling, and swimming. These exercises increase the flow of blood to your working muscles. Exercising muscles receive as much as 20 times the blood flow of resting muscles.

Other Ways to Relax

Many people develop their own ways to relax. Some find that short naps help. Others have asked whether the use of tranquilizers to combat stress would lower blood pressure. Tranquilizers don't really lower blood pressure and should not be used for that purpose.

> I seem to have taught myself my own method. I simply let my mind go blank. Rather than argue with the children, who don't hear me anyway, I realized that at some point, I'd just end up hurting myself. So, during tense times, I stare out the window and go blank. However you do it, it helps. —Louise M.

SUMMARY

Any or several of the alternatives to drug therapy may be effective in lowering blood pressure for certain individuals, but they are seldom the only answer. Many people who lose weight can't keep it off. If they gain weight again, their blood pressure is likely to rise. A very low-salt diet is quite hard to stick to, although a modest reduction in salt is often helpful. To be useful, relaxation techniques have to be practiced regularly. And, while exercise is probably good for your cardiovascular system, its effect on lowering blood pressure is usually slight. However, the goal of therapy is to reduce and control your blood pressure—it doesn't matter how you do it. So, if these methods appeal to you, try them.

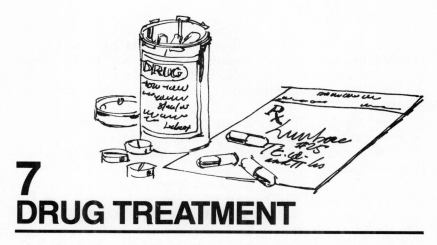

7
DRUG TREATMENT

The drugs used to control hypertension work by making adjustments in one or more of the mechanisms that regulate blood pressure. There are many drugs currently in use, and more are being developed all the time. Different ones have different purposes, and some work better in some people than in other people. Some people need a combination of two or more medications. And, the amount of a particular drug that any individual needs will vary from person to person.

So, the early stage of treatment is like a trial-and-error period, as you and your doctor try different dosages and combinations of drugs to find what works best for you. During this time, your schedule of drugs may change often, which can be confusing.

A SERIOUS PROBLEM

A serious problem in treating high blood pressure is that many people—estimates range from 20 to perhaps 50 percent—simply stop taking or never start taking drugs that have been prescribed. Let's look at why some people are tempted to stop taking their medicine:

• Most people with hypertension don't feel sick. Therefore, they don't believe that they need medication, or they take it only when they don't feel well. Some people have trouble accepting the fact that they have a medical problem.
• A lot of people don't understand that high blood pressure is a serious problem if it is *not* treated.

Taking pills to prevent illness was a hard thing to understand
at first.   —Nancy L.

47

• Since drugs for high blood pressure often have side effects, people don't want to trade feeling well for feeling poorly. Some people don't know that if a side effect is troublesome, the chances are that a different medicine or a lower dosage will not cause that problem.

• Once their blood pressure is lowered, some people mistakenly think that they are cured and no longer need the medicine.

• Some are discouraged by the fact that they may have to take drugs indefinitely.

• Some people don't like drugs in general and therefore subconsciously "forget" to take theirs. Then, if they don't feel any different, they may deliberately stop taking them.

• Some people may have other medical conditions as well, and if they feel poorly, they may blame it on the medicine for high blood pressure.

• Because they believe that hypertension affects only people who are nervous and tense, some people don't take their pills unless they're feeling nervous or tense.

• So many different drugs have been prescribed that people get confused.

• The scheduled times are not convenient.

• The medicine is too expensive.

• They simply forget and no one helps remind them.

• They are afraid of becoming dependent on the drug.

> I have a lot of patients who think they know when their blood pressure is up. They only take their medicine then. You cannot tell when your pressure is up, and you've got to take the medicine regularly. —Dr. B.

As we have said, though, most of you will need to take one or more medicines. The chances are good that they will be successful in lowering your blood pressure. But they must also be taken after your pressure is down, to keep it down. Therefore, if you are tempted to stop for any reason—talk it over with your doctor. Your doctor will be glad that you really want to succeed.

USING PRESCRIPTION DRUGS

Prescription drugs play a major role in modern medicine, but the subject of drugs and their proper use can be complicated. And it's easy to understand why. For example, different drugs can be used for the same purpose, or the same drug may go by different names. As another example, every drug has its own *regimen*—that is, when and how it should be taken—which can be especially confusing if you need more than one.

We believe that you will find drug-taking easier if you understand *why* you should take your drugs and *how* they work to lower your blood pressure. This is particularly true for hypertension, because you may be taking several, each one with a different purpose. You may be told to increase or decrease the amount of a certain drug for various reasons, such as if you have a cold or plan on heavy exercise. You will need to know which drugs do what.

In the following, we talk first about prescription drugs in general, to help you understand why the proper use of medications is so important. Later on, we give information on the drugs most commonly prescribed for high blood pressure and discuss some of their specific modes of action.

What You Should Know about Your Medicines

Whenever a drug is prescribed for you, you should know:
- Its name.
- Why you are taking it—that is, what it does.
- When and how often you should take it.
- How much of it you should take.
- Whether it has any serious side effects and what you should do if they occur.
- Whether it will interfere with any other drugs that you may be taking.
- Whether you must be careful about drinking alcohol or need to avoid certain activities such as driving.

Following Your Regimen: When and How Much

It's important to take a drug at the *times* and in the *amount* specified. The *dosage* prescribed is the amount that your doctor thinks *you* need; other patients with high blood pressure may need more or less than you do.

Some drugs don't work well unless the full amount is taken. It can also be dangerous to take more than the amount prescribed. Never stop your medication unless you are told to. For certain drugs, problems can develop if you stop them suddenly. And for high blood pressure, if you stop your medicine, your pressure will just go up again.

Some drugs are absorbed into your system better if they are taken with food; others work best in an empty stomach. Be sure you know *when* you should take your medicine and *with what*. If the instructions aren't fully clear, ask. For instance, what if your prescription says "take before meals" but you usually skip breakfast?

Also find out whether there are times that you should *not* take a dose. Some medicines should not be taken if you have a cold or are ill. Others should not be taken before driving or heavy exercise or after drinking alcoholic beverages. Some medications may need to be restarted in a particular way in order to prevent problems.

Ask your doctor what you should do if you forget a pill or if you take too many. Everybody forgets to take pills once in a while. If this should happen, don't be embarrassed to admit it. Your doctor *needs* this information to tell whether the drug is working for you.

If you have trouble remembering to take your medicine at the scheduled times—or have many drugs, all to be taken at different times—ask your doctor or druggist to help you figure out a more convenient schedule. We talk more about ways to remember your pills in Chapter 8.

> I keep my pills beside my toothbrush, so I rarely forget.
> —Nancy L.

Other Precautions

In prescribing a drug for you, your doctor will also need to know other facts, such as whether you have any allergies, have previously had bad reactions to medicine, or are on a special diet. Some drugs can be harmful if you are pregnant or nursing or if you may become pregnant. Again, ask your doctor if this applies to you.

Some people worry about becoming physically or emotionally dependent on prescribed drugs. Most drugs given for specific illnesses or medical conditions are not habit-forming. If you are concerned, ask your doctor about yours.

Whenever you are given a new drug, ask your doctor whether it will make you feel any different. Find out whether any side effects will interfere with your normal activities. For example, if a drug is likely to make you dizzy or sleepy, perhaps you shouldn't drive a car or operate heavy machinery after taking it. Or, maybe you should take it after the activity. Particular problems that sometimes occur with medicine for high blood pressure are discussed later in this chapter.

Keeping Track of Your Medicines

If you are seeing more than one doctor, make sure that all of them know exactly what drugs you are taking. This includes your dentist, too. Some drugs, including birth control pills, should not be taken in combination with certain others. Thus, it is extremely important that your doctor know all the other medicines that you may be taking, even things that you can buy without a prescription, like aspirin or cold remedies. It may be helpful to make a list of your drugs or even take the bottles with you when you go to the doctor's.

(Actually, if you are seeing more than one doctor, all of them should know that, too. This may be hard to admit, especially if you are afraid of "hurting the other doc's feelings," but it really is important. Not only can certain drugs interact harmfully, but so can other medical treatment and advice.)

Storing Medicines

Some medicines have special storage instructions, such as keeping them in the refrigerator or away from sunlight. Others require a dry place, which may rule out the bathroom. Your pharmacist can advise you on these points.

Since moisture, even from your hands, can make some pills lose their effectiveness, simply pour a few into the bottle cap rather than into your hand to pick one out.

Some Safety Tips About All Drugs

Finally, because the wrong medicine in the wrong person can be extremely dangerous, a few rules should be followed for safety's sake:

- Throw out drugs that are older than the *expiration date* on the label. They may have changed with age. Ask your doctor or pharmacist whether you should also toss out drugs that you no longer need.
- When you throw away drugs, flush them down the toilet. Don't throw them into a wastebasket where someone else may find them.
- Keep drugs out of the reach of children.
- If you have trouble opening the child-proof caps required by law, and if there are no children in the house, ask the pharmacist to use different caps.
- Never take someone else's medicine, even if your illnesses are the same. Likewise, never give someone else your medicine.
- Keep the labels on the bottles so that you always know what is in the bottles.
- If you think you took too many pills or if a child got into

them, call your doctor, pharmacist, or poison control center immediately. Keep their phone numbers by the telephone.

DRUGS FOR HIGH BLOOD PRESSURE

A wide variety of drugs are used to lower blood pressure. They work on many different parts of the body's complicated blood pressure regulation system. Appendix III, p. 73, lists the drugs most frequently used today so that you can see how many your doctor has to choose from. They are given by their *generic* (or common) name and by their brand names. New medicines are constantly being introduced. If your medicine doesn't appear on the list, that may be why. Ask your doctor if you are curious.

Diuretics

The most commonly prescribed drugs for high blood pressure are *diuretics,* often called "water pills" or "fluid pills." They lower the pressure in the blood vessels by washing excess salt and water from the body. This reduces the amount of fluid circulating in the bloodstream, which reduces the pressure in the arteries.

As the diuretic begins to wash fluid from your body, you will probably notice an increase in how often you need to urinate, at least for a few days. Because of this, it makes sense not to take a diuretic after about 6 p.m., so you won't have to get up in the middle of the night. In addition, diuretics sometimes cause too much fluid to be lost, especially in hot weather. Check with your doctor if you should feel ill or faint. As a rule, low dosages of diuretics rarely cause symptoms, but recent studies suggest the need for reassessing the role of these drugs. For instance, a diuretic may increase cholesterol levels and decrease body potassium levels. Such chemical changes may counter-balance the benefit received from the lowered blood pressure achieved by the diuretic. These changes do not occur in all patients being treated with diuretics, but they may develop over a long period of time. Therefore, your doctor may wish to monitor your cholesterol and potassium levels while you are taking diuretics. If he finds that these levels are out of the normal range, your doctor may choose an alternate drug to reduce your blood pressure, or he may take other steps to control your cholesterol and potassium levels while keeping you on the diuretic.

While all diuretics basically do the same job, there are differences in how strong they are and how fast they work. In most cases, diuretics called *thiazides* are tried first. The thiazides are fairly mild. Their major problem is that some of them cause the loss of too much potassium.

Other drugs are also used in treating high blood pressure, either alone or in addition to a diuretic. The diuretic helps make the other types work better, so that smaller doses of each are needed.

Sympatholytics

Another group of drugs, called sympatholytics, acts on different parts of the sympathetic nervous system to lower blood pressure. Some of these work by reducing the amount of blood the heart pumps with each beat as well as reducing the heart rate. Others relax the blood vessels indirectly by blocking nervous system signals that cause them to tighten up or contract. When the arterioles contract, blood pressure increases. So, by preventing contraction, these drugs reduce the pressure. When a drug is needed in addition to a diuretic, a sympatholytic is usually tried first.

Vasodilators

A third group, called vasodilators, works by relaxing the blood vessels directly. These drugs cause the muscular walls of the blood vessels (*vaso-*) to widen (*dilate*), which lowers the pressure in them.

Converting Enzyme Inhibitors

The newest group of drugs for high blood pressure is called *converting enzyme inhibitors*. They inhibit or reduce the production of angiotensin, a substance in the body that is involved in regulating blood pressure.

Blood Pressure Drugs and Side Effects

Most drugs prescribed for hypertension produce some side effects, although many of them are minor and not even noticeable. However, because side effects are responsible for some people dropping out of treatment, we discuss some of the more common problems here.

Keep in mind that *nobody* gets all the side effects that we or anybody else might mention. Many people never get any. Also, two or more drugs are often prescribed for hypertension, and the combination may affect your body in a very different way from either drug alone. Ask your doctor what *you* might expect from your medicine.

> People don't really end up having as many side effects as some lists suggest. It is useful to know what *might* happen, but a lot of people don't have any bad effects from their medicine.
> —Dr. W.

When starting a new drug, you will need patience for a while. Many side effects disappear within a few days, once your body gets used to the new medicine. But if they don't go away, adjustments can usually be made. For example, some problems are related to the amount of the drug taken, so a lower dosage may be tried. Or a different drug may be better. Sometimes an additional drug can be prescribed to counteract the side effects. As you can see from the lengthy list of drugs later in this chapter, many medicines are available; surely, one of them will work for you.

> The drug I was taking used to make me tired all the time. The doctor discontinued it and gave me another one. I feel better now. —Debra S.

One particular problem is encountered with several drugs for hypertension. *Orthostatic* or *postural hypotension (hypo*tension means *low* blood pressure) is the name given to a condition that may produce a dizzy or woozy feeling if you get up suddenly after sitting or lying down. The room may seem to go around for a few seconds. Occasionally it can cause fainting. It may go away after your body adjusts to the drug, but in some cases, it never disappears completely. If you sit for a minute or so before getting up, the dizziness should not be a problem. If it becomes troublesome, mention it. Certain exercises may be helpful.

You should also be aware that most drugs used for hypertension interact with alcohol. In particular, alcohol tends to make orthostatic hypotension worse. Check specifically about the drugs that have been prescribed for you.

Other fairly common side effects may also occur. They are usually minor and temporary, disappearing after a few days. For example, some drugs may cause tiredness at first or a dry mouth or stuffy nose. More troublesome problems related to medicines used for hypertension include unusual mood changes, depression, muscle pains or cramps in the legs, and swelling in the feet and lower legs. Some people experience sexual problems, such as lack of desire or impotence. If any of these or anything else should continue to bother you, don't hesitate to talk about it with your physician. For most people, there is a solution.

> I first found out about my high blood pressure 10 years ago. I started treatment, but the drugs interfered with my sexual feelings, so I stopped. Later, I went somewhere else and got different drugs. But they made me jittery, made by mouth dry, and gave me nightmares, so I stopped them, too. A few months ago, I started treatment again using a different medicine, and so far, I'm doing all right. —Nathan R.

All medicines may not produce the same effects in different people. Your doctor needs to know how yours acts in your body. Therefore, while you should be patient and allow your body to get used to the medicine you should also report all symptoms or side effects, even things that you think are minor. Some problems may be uncomfortable enough that you should call the doctor as soon as you notice them. Less troublesome problems can probably wait until your next office visit. But if there is any real change in the way you feel, let your doctor help you figure out the reason. While some problems may be related to the drug, others may be caused by something else. All this information is important.

In the past, doctors were often reluctant to mention possible side effects. They were afraid that the suggestion of, for example, dizziness, would *cause* people to feel dizzy. Today, they are much more aware that side effects can be a real concern. At the same time, some people feel embarrassed talking about side effects. Some, in an effort to please, want to give a good report or don't want to fuss. But your doctor needs to know how *your* drug makes *you* feel.

Occasionally, however, a side effect may remain. If a drug agrees with you in other ways and works well, you may have to learn to live with a certain side effect. The goal is to keep side effects to a minimum.

Several drugs used for hypertension may affect other medical conditions or may interact with drugs taken for such conditions. For example, some drugs may interfere with a treatment for diabetes or asthma. Even previous medical conditions, such as depression and ulcers, can be affected. Your doctor, of course, should be told about any present or past medical problem, as well as any other medication that you may be taking now. This information can make a difference in choosing the best medicine for your high blood pressure.

Finding the Right Combination

Although we called the early stage "trial and error," drug therapy is not really guesswork. Your doctor doesn't just pull a drug out of a hat and give it to you. Treatment usually follows a logical sequence of phases, with a particular goal at each one. Therapy is individualized for each person, so that you will end up with as few drugs and as low a dosage as possible.

Doctors usually begin with a small dosage of a single drug. Either the dosage or the type of drug will be changed if the blood pressure goal is not reached at each stage. First, a higher dosage might be tried; then a second drug would be added or substituted if necessary, and so on, until the desired drop in blood pressure is achieved and the serious side effects are eliminated.

> My pressure slips upward every once in a while. When that happens, the dosage is increased or a new drug is added.
> —Paul W.

After your blood pressure has been lowered and is under control, a few other medication changes may be made that can make your schedule more convenient. Many drugs for high blood pressure are combined in *fixed dosages* into a single tablet or capsule. If the exact combination that you need exists in such a *combination drug*, you may be able to switch to it. A fixed-dose combination is usually not prescribed until the individual ingredients have been tried successfully first. The names of the combination drugs in use today are listed in Appendix III, p. 75.

> If you work with your doctor until you get the right medicine for you, you *will* find one. There are a lot of medicines out there.
> —Nathan R.

Medications and Diet

Depending on your treatment program, some changes in your diet may be necessary. Your doctor will give you specific dietary instructions if appropriate.

For example, some restriction of salt is often advised for people with high blood pressure, but it is especially important for those taking diuretics. One of the jobs of a diuretic is to get rid of excess sodium. By reducing salt in the diet, the drug works better. In fact, if you eat a great deal of salt (more than 2 teaspoons a day), the diuretic won't be effective.

Also, as we explained earlier, some diuretics cause potassium to be washed out of the body. Other diuretics cause potassium to be retained. Most people can get along with a slightly low or slightly high level of potassium, but very low or very high levels can cause problems. Your doctor may check the level of potassium in your blood from time to time. If it is too low, a potassium-retaining diuretic may be prescribed. You may need to make changes in your diet or take a potassium supplement. Foods that are high in potassium are listed in Appendix II, p. 69, together with some information about potassium supplements. Again, a dietitian can supply you with more complete information. Note also that some salt substitutes contain potassium; check with your doctor before using one. (See Appendix I, no. 6, p.68).

Some medications may cause your blood fat (cholesterol) levels to rise. Since high cholesterol is another important risk factor for heart disease, your physician may check your cholesterol levels occasionally. If it seems too high, he may switch you to another drug, one which doesn't raise cholesterol, or he may instruct you to follow a low-cholesterol diet.

These adjustments in your eating habits may not be as complicated as they sound. Furthermore, many goals can be accomplished at once by a few dietary changes.

Other Considerations

Costs. Drug-taking for high blood pressure can sometimes be expensive, although the cost is usually less than $1 a day. However, you can't afford *not* to take your drugs. Drugs are much cheaper than a disability caused by untreated hypertension, which might involve a hospital stay and lost income. If cost is a problem, talk it over with your doctor.

The prices of drugs vary, depending on which drug is prescribed, how many doses are prescribed, and where you buy the medicine. You may want to discuss these matters with your doctor and pharmacist.

Although you might be able to save money by comparing prices among drugstores, it may also be wise to pick out a convenient drugstore and stick with it. This is especially true if more than one doctor is prescribing drugs for you. A pharmacist who knows you can help keep track of your medicines, including drugs that you can buy without a prescription, and can warn you if one of them may interact badly with another one. Your pharmacist may also be able to help you figure out a schedule for taking your medicines or advise you on the possibilities of buying in bulk or other ways to cut costs.

Taking Other Medicines. Several medicines that you can buy without a prescription, such as cold remedies, nasal sprays and inhalers, laxatives, and antacids, can interfere with your blood pressure control. Some contain sodium and may undo the work of a diuretic; others may counteract the drugs you are taking to relax your blood vessels. Diet pills and asthma medications may also be harmful, depending on your blood pressure medicine. Some medicines have warnings on the label not to take them if you have high blood pressure. Others list their ingredients, and you should avoid those that contain sodium. However, since not all medicines give ingredients or warnings, *you should check with your doctor or pharmacist before taking anything other than what has been prescribed.*

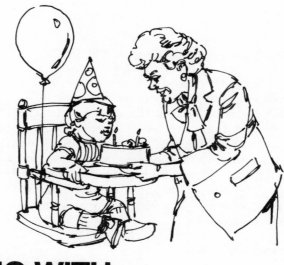

8
LIVING WITH HYPERTENSION

In some ways, high blood pressure is a very complicated condition, and in other ways, it is simple. The complicated parts include how and why the condition develops, what can happen if it is not treated, and the many kinds and combinations of drugs used to treat it. These things are hard to explain, and even medical experts don't yet understand everything there is to know about high blood pressure. The simple part is that you don't *have* to understand all the complexities to follow your treatment. The main things needed on your part are to:

- Accept the fact that you have high blood pressure.
- Decide to get the benefits of controlling it.
- Visit your doctor regularly to have your blood pressure checked.
- Take your drugs as prescribed.
- Keep your doctor informed.

However, controlling high blood pressure is a long-term project, and we believe that you can help manage your health better if you take an active interest in your condition. By trying to understand more about hypertension, we think that you will find living with it much easier.

> After I was hospitalized following the hemorrhage in my eye, everybody was so worried about me that no one bothered to "educate" me. There's a lot I still want to learn. —Debra S.

FINDING THE RIGHT TREATMENT PROGRAM

The short-term goal of treatment is to lower your blood pressure and to keep it under control. Fortunately, there are many ways that this can be done, so the second part of the goal is to do so with a minimum number of side effects, at minimum cost, and with maximum comfort. The vast majority of people with hypertension are able to control their blood pressure well and easily with a simple combination of a few drugs. Upon reaching this goal you go a long way toward the ultimate objective of preventing the complications of untreated hypertension; including coronary heart disease, stroke, and kidney damage.

Working with Your Doctor

Just as you may have personal preferences about your lifestyle and treatment options, your doctor, too, may have preferences about the way high blood pressure should be treated. For example, some doctors have people with mild hypertension try dieting or salt reduction first; they will then prescribe drugs if that doesn't work. Other doctors prefer to prescribe drugs first and also suggest, for example, weight loss.

> Fear of serious complications needn't be the only reason for following therapy. Some patients take their medicine faithfully simply to please the doctor or family or to get their life insurance rates lowered. At least I know that with their blood pressure down, they're helping themselves to live longer and healthier. —Dr. M.

In the long run, regardless of your doctor's particular approach, we believe that it is essential for you and your doctor to have a good relationship, so that you can work out a treatment program that suits you both. Effective treatment for any condition depends in part on both of you agreeing on the same course of action, which can happen only when you understand the goals of treatment. Be sure that your doctor explains things clearly to you, in terms that you understand. Don't hesitate to ask questions, no matter how minor or silly you think they are.

> For some people, information on diet and stress is too confusing. They need a doctor to help sort it all out. —Benjamin B.

> I can ask my doctor anything. At first, though, I didn't ask many questions because I think I was nervous about hearing the answers. I simply trusted my doctor. —Nancy L.

Follow-Up Visits

Once your blood pressure has been lowered, you'll still need to visit the doctor every few months, but things should settle into a fairly comfortable routine. Your medication schedule won't change as often, after the right combination of therapy has been found. However, over the years, other changes in your health and life may mean that you need less or more of a drug or a different drug. Sometimes you may require only a temporary change in medications—for example, if you are going through a period of stress. And, of course, new and better drugs are always under development. So your doctor will keep watch on your prescriptions and make changes as necessary.

> I see my doctor every three months. I respect what he knows about my health. My only health plan is to enjoy myself—that's why I need to do what he tells me.   —Benjamin B.

These follow-up visits are very important to make sure that your blood pressure stays down. If you have to cancel an appointment for any reason, make another one right away. Since you probably feel fine, it's easy to forget an appointment or put off calling for one.

WORKING OUT PROBLEMS

If you decide to make a change in your lifestyle to help your high blood pressure or to control another risk factor for cardiovascular disease, be sure that you understand why the change may be helpful. You should also believe that the change can make a difference. If too many changes are imposed, some people are inclined to stop *all* treatment.

If you have difficulty making a change, ask for assistance. For example, if you need to lose a large amount of weight and have trouble sticking to your diet, get help in planning one that you can live with. Otherwise, it simply won't work, you'll get discouraged, and you may give up.

Living with hypertension can be tedious, especially at first, but in the long run, it needn't be complicated, costly, or uncomfortable. If it is, discuss the difficulties with your doctor. Most people simply don't like having to follow an indefinite treatment program, and most doctors understand how hard it is.

You and your doctor should also set up some ground rules

on when to call, what symptoms to report, and what to do if either the doctor or you are away.

REMEMBERING TO TAKE YOUR PILLS

Making a Schedule

Your doctor, of course, will keep records of your progress. But you may want to, also. You may also want to keep a diary on how you feel. Take it with you on your next office visit, and let the doctor help you figure out whether a side effect or other symptom is related to a drug.

Diaries such as these can be very helpful to both you and your doctor, especially during the early stages. They can also be useful in planning how to make drug-taking easier. If your medicine says "take every 6 hours," does that mean in the middle of the night, too? What if early morning is typically so hectic that you keep forgetting a pill? Do you work nights? Do you travel a lot? By looking at your drug schedule and thinking about your normal routine, you and your doctor can work out a schedule that is con-venient for you. Pharmacists and nurses can be helpful here, too. You may also want to make a note of what (or who) reminds you to take your pills.

Planning Makes It Easier

It's very easy to get confused—and even annoyed—if you have a lot of different medicines, all to be taken at different times. Most drugstores carry special pill containers with separate compartments for each day of the week, which you may find helpful.

Some people find it helpful to make a chart showing when they should take their medicines. Some people draw a clock face, with a picture and the name of each pill next to the times they should take them. Others keep their schedule on a blackboard or tape notes to themselves on the refrigerator or the bathroom mirror. Do what-ever will help you remember.

As much as possible, try to work your medicines into some part of your everyday routine, such as when you wash up in the morning, at meals, or when getting ready for bed. It may also be useful to keep all your medicines in a particular place that you can't overlook, such as on the kitchen table. Wherever you decide to keep them, make sure that they are out of the reach of young children.

I keep some at work, too, in case I forget my morning pill.
—Nancy L.

Plan Ahead

If you're going away, expecting visitors, or doing anything out of your normal routine, plan ahead. Be sure that you always have enough of all your medicines. Also, particularly if you'll be on vacation or away from home, refill your prescriptions before you run out—so that you won't run out. If you plan to travel by plane, carry your medicines with you; don't check them with your luggage.

MEASURING YOUR BLOOD PRESSURE AT HOME

Sometimes It's Helpful

Some doctors have their patients measure their own blood pressure at home. This may be especially helpful during the early stage, when your doctor wants to know how much your pressure varies during the day or how your body reacts to certain medications. Some people are encouraged to continue this monitoring after a treatment program has been established. This can reassure them that their medicines are working and may help make it easier to keep taking drugs even when they feel well.

> My husband takes my pressure regularly. My doctor didn't suggest it but was glad to hear that I had a sphygmomanometer. It relieves a lot of worry on my part. Sometimes when I think my pressure is up, it isn't. But if it is, I lie down for a while and it goes down again.   —Debra S.

Sometimes It's Not

On the other hand, most doctors don't believe that home monitoring is necessary. Some people become anxious when they take their blood pressure often, and they may overreact to its natural ups and downs during the day. Some may even try to adjust their medications according to their blood pressure, which can be dangerous.

> Once I used a machine at the drugstore, and it showed such a high pressure that I went straight to the clinic without an appointment. I was really scared. The clinic said I was fine and to forget it, so I stay away from those things now.
> —Benjamin B.

If You Take Your Blood Pressure

If you decide to monitor your own blood pressure, take it on the same arm each time, and in the same body position, generally while sitting. It is a good idea to record what you were doing immediately before you took it—for example, following a hectic day at work, scrubbing the floors, or reading.

If you take your own blood pressure, you will need to find out which blood pressure reading indicates that you should call your doctor. Sometimes the doctor may be able to adjust your medicines over the phone. Occasionally, by sending your readings to your doctor every month or so, the number of office visits may be reduced.

Several kits are available for measuring blood pressure. They vary a lot in both price and accuracy. Your doctor or local chapter of the American Heart Association may be able to recommend one. Most come with directions, but the best way to learn is by watching someone do it and by practicing. Ask your doctor or nurse to teach you. If you do buy a kit, make sure you check its accuracy every so often by comparing it with the one in your doctor's office.

OTHER THINGS TO CONSIDER

Working with Your Family

Some families, as well as some patients, overreact to having high blood pressure and think that their whole lives will have to change. If your family members seem overly concerned, have them visit your doctor with you for reassurance. Also, since hypertension tends to run in families, other members may want to find out about their own risk factors. In particular, if you have a daughter who is taking birth control pills or some form of *estrogen* hormone, be sure that she has her blood pressure checked every 6 months. Birth control pills and estrogens have been linked with hypertension.

It probably makes sense for all people, with or without high blood pressure, to watch their weight, cut down on salt, and try to find a means of relieving stress. But this is particularly true for your children. Childhood is the time to set healthy patterns. If your children get used to good eating and lifestyle habits, they may not have to struggle to make changes later on in life. At the least, have their blood pressure checked every year.

Life Insurance

Life insurance rates are usually higher for people with hypertension, and some people are not able to get life insurance at all. If this is your case, tell your insurance company as soon as you are under a doctor's care, and keep the company informed of your progress. When your blood pressure has come down, you may be able to get your costs reduced, and the rates may decrease even more after you have been in treatment for several years.

SUCCESS AND YOU

With only a few exceptions, high blood pressure can be lowered and kept under control quite successfully. And it can be done without major changes or discomfort. *The most important ingredient for success is you.* To succeed, you need to believe that your health is important and that the benefits of treatment outweigh the costs and difficulties.

We realize that "health" is not necessarily your first priority every day, so we like to think in terms of love of life, as well as love of health.

> I never forget my pills because I love me! I get a good feeling when I do something for my health.   —Benjamin B.

APPENDIX I

1. Your local chapter of the American Heart Association can provide the following publications on dietary fats: *Cholesterol and Your Heart* (1984); *Nutrition Labeling: Food Selection Hints for Fat Controlled Meals* (Rev. 1982); *Recipes for Fat Controlled Low Cholesterol Meals from the American Heart Association Cookbooks* (Rev. 1981).

2. An excellent booklet on losing weight, *Are You Really Serious About Losing Weight?*, is available through your doctor from Pennwalt Corporation, P. O. Box 1766, Rochester, New York 14603. The information is updated regularly to include the latest on weight loss in general and on special diets for people with heart disease, high blood pressure, and diabetes. The 84-page booklet contains realistic and encouraging advice plus many useful charts and tables.

3. *The Sodium Content of Your Food,* by A. C. Marsh, R. N. Klippstein, and S. D. Kaplan, United States Department of Agriculture, Home and Garden Bulletin Number 233, U. S. Government Printing Office, Washington, DC 20402 ($2.25). This book contains one of the best lists of sodium content in foods and certain medicines.

4. *Your 500 Milligram Sodium Diet, Your 1000 Milligram Sodium Diet,* and *Your Mild Sodium-Restricted Diet* are available with a doctor's note from the American Heart Association, 44 East 23rd Street, New York, New York 10010, or from a local American Heart Association chapter. These small books are full of useful, realistic suggestions and advice on achieving different levels of sodium restriction. Information includes, for example, how to plan a diet with regard to both salt and calories, tips for the cook, and tips on eating out. Sample menus are given for different numbers of calories. Condensed versions are also available.

   How to Live 365 Days a Year the Salt-Free Way, by J. P. Brunswick, D. Love, and A. Weinberg, Bantam Books, New York, 1977 ($2.50). The food charts, which list sodium, potassium and calorie content, are extensive and include many low-sodium products.

Nutrition for the Prime of Your Life, by Annette Natow and Jo-Ann Hestin, McGraw-Hill, 1983 ($8.95, paperback).

5. *Beyond Diet—Exercise Your Way to Fitness and Heart Health,* by L. R. Zohman, is an excellent booklet available from Best Foods Nutrition Service, Box 307, Coventry, Connecticut 06238.

6. *Facts about Potassium,* a pamphlet available from the American Heart Association, lists the sodium content and calories in potassium-rich foods.

APPENDIX II

SAMPLE HIGH- AND LOW-SODIUM MENUS*

HIGH IN SODIUM		LOW IN SODIUM	
Breakfast			
1 cup cocoa, from dry mix	232 mg	1 cup orange juice	5mg
¾ cup instant oatmeal with maple and brown sugar	277 mg	1 cup puffed wheat or rice cereal	1 gm
		½ cup milk	60 mg
1 slice Canadian bacon	394 mg	banana	2 mg
1 slice toast with butter	230 mg	cinnamon sweet roll, frozen	110 mg
Lunch			
1 fish sandwich (fast food)	882 mg	1 peanut butter sandwich on white bread	309 mg
1 dill pickle	928 mg	apple	2 mg
10 potato chips	200 mg	1 cup yogurt with fruit	133 mg
Dinner			
3 oz. ham	1114 mg	3 oz. pork chop	60 mg
1 cup mashed potatoes, instant	485 mg	baked potato	5 mg
with butter	116 mg	with sour cream	12 mg
½ cup canned spinach	455 mg	3 oz. frozen spinach	65 mg
salad with 1 Tbsp. French dressing, bottled	214 mg	salad with 1 Tbsp. French dressing, home recipe	92 mg
½ cup chocolate pudding, instant	470 mg	1 slice frozen banana cream pie	90 mg
(before adding salt)	5997 mg	(before adding salt)	946 mg

*Sodium is measured in *milligrams*, abbreviated *mg*. One thousand milligrams equals 1 gram, or about one-fifth teaspoon. See Appendix I, no. 3, p. 67 for the source of the sodium values given here and in the following list.

(continues on next page)

(continued from previous page)

SODIUM CONTENT OF SELECTED FOODS

HIGHER IN SODIUM		LOWER IN SODIUM	
5 oz. chicken, canned	714 mg	7 oz. chicken, roasted	138 mg
Big Mac	1510 mg	hamburger, bun, lettuce and tomato, homemade	200 mg
2 oz. dried beef	2440 mg	3 oz. fresh beef	55 mg
3 oz. shrimp, canned	1955 mg	3 oz. shrimp, fresh	137 mg
2 frankfurters	1278 mg	3 oz. haddock	150 mg
meatloaf TV dinner	1304 mg	Swiss steak TV dinner	682 mg
turkey pot pie, frozen	1018 mg	turkey pot pie, homemade	620 mg
1 cup vegetable beef soup from dry mix	1000 mg	1 cup vegetable beef soup, low sodium	51 mg
1 cup canned tomato soup	932 mg	1 cup canned tomato soup, low sodium	29 mg
1 cup canned split pea soup	987 mg	1 cup dried split peas	5 mg
1 cup kidney beans, canned	844 mg	1 cup dried kidney beans	4 mg
1 cup beets, canned	479 mg	1 cup broccoli, frozen	35 mg
½ cup mushrooms, canned	484 mg	1 cup mushrooms, raw	7 mg
1 cup sauerkraut	1554 mg	1 cup cabbage, raw	8 mg
1 cup carrots, canned	386 mg	1 carrot, raw	34 mg
1 cup creamed corn, canned	671 mg	2 ears corn on the cob	2 mg
1 cup tomatoes, canned	390 mg	2 tomatoes, raw	28 mg

HIGHER IN SODIUM		LOWER IN SODIUM	
1 dill pickle	928 mg	1 cucumber	14 mg
1 cup vegetable juice cocktail	887 mg	1 cup apple cider	5 mg
4 green olives	323 mg	3 black olives	96 mg
1 Tbsp. soy sauce	1029 mg	1 Tbsp. catsup	156 mg
1 Tbsp. butter, salted	116 mg	1 Tbsp. butter, unsalted	2 mg
1 oz. American cheese	406 mg	1 oz. cheddar cheese	176 mg
4 oz. cottage cheese	457 mg	4 oz. cottage cheese, unsalted	14 mg
1 cup Rice Krispies	340 mg	1 cup puffed rice	1 mg
1 cup Wheaties	355 mg	1 biscuit Shredded Wheat	3 mg
1 biscuit from mix	272 mg	1 brown and serve roll	138 mg
1 cup stuffing mix, cooked	1131 mg	1 cup noodles, cooked	2 mg

POTASSIUM AND POTASSIUM SUPPLEMENTS

Some Foods That Are High In Potassium

bananas	potatoes	chicken
orange juice	flounder	soybeans
melons	broccoli	molasses
grapefruit juice	raisins	nectarines
prune juice	strawberries	spinach
avocados	squash	veal

(continues on next page)

(continued from previous page)

POTASSIUM SUPPLEMENTS

Brand Names: Slow-K, Kay-Ciel, K-Lor, Kaon, Pfiklor, and several others

Form: Liquid, tablet, or powder

How to take: With or following foods. When taken on an empty stomach, potassium can have a mild laxative effect or cause an upset stomach.

Precautions: Let your doctor know immediately if you have stomach pain and indigestion or if you notice blackish stools or other signs of intestinal bleeding. If you have trouble swallowing the tablets, tell the doctor.

Note: Potassium supplements should not be used unless recommended by your doctor. They can be dangerous if you have certain kidney problems or are using potassium-retaining diuretics.

APPENDIX III

COMMON DRUGS USED FOR HYPERTENSION

Common or
generic names

Some commonly used
brand names

DIURETICS

Thiazide diuretics

bendroflumethiazide	Naturetin
benzthiazide	Aquatag, Exna, Hydrex
chlorothiazide	Diuril, SK-Chlorothiazide
chlorthalidone	Hygroton, Thalitone
cyclothiazide	Anhydron, Fluidil
hydrochlorothiazide	Esidrix, HydroDiuril, Oretic
hydroflumethiazide	Diucardin, Saluron
indapamide	Lozol
methyclothiazide	Aquatensen, Enduron
metolazone	Diulo, Zaroxolyn
polythiazide	Renese
quinethazone	Hydromox
trichlormethiazide	Metahydrin, Naqua

Loop diuretics

bumetanide	Bumex
ethacrynic acid	Edecrin
furosemide	Lasix

Potassium-retaining diuretics

amiloride	Midamor
spironolactone	Aldactone
triamterene	Dyrenium

(continues on next page)

(continued from previous page)

SYMPATHOLYTICS

atenolol	Tenormin
clonidine	Catapres
guanabenz	Wytensin
guanadrel	Hylorel
guanethidine	Ismelin
labetalol	Trandate, Normodyne
methyldopa	Aldomet
metoprolol	Lopressor
nadolol	Corgard
oxprenolol	Trasicor
pindolol	Visken
prazosin	Minipress
propranolol	Inderal, Inderal LA
reserpine and rauwolfia alkaloids	Harmonyl, Raudixin, Rau–Sed Sandril, Serpasil
timolol	Blocadren

VASODILATORS

hydralazine	Apresoline, Dralzine
minoxidil	Loniten

CONVERTING ENZYME INHIBITORS

captopril	Capoten

APPENDIX III (continued)

COMBINATION MEDICINES

Brand Names	**Common or generic names**
Aldactazide	hydrochlorothiazide & spironolactone
Aldoclor	chlorothiazide & methyldopa
Aldoril	hydrochlorothiazide & methyldopa
Apresazide	hydrochlorothiazide & hydralazine
Apresodex	hydrochlorothiazide & hydralazine
Apresoline-Esidrix	hydrochlorothiazide & hydralazine
Capozide	hydrochlorothiazide & captopril
Combipres	chlorthalidone & clonidine
Corzide	bendroflumethiazide & nadolol
Demi-Regroton	chlorthalidone & reserpine
Diupres	chlorothiazide & reserpine
Diutensen-R	methyclothiazide & reserpine
Dyazide	hydrochlorothiazide & triamterene
Enduronyl	methyclothiazide & reserpine
Esimil	hydrochlorothiazide & guanethidine
Exna-R	benzthiazide & reserpine
Hydral	hydrochlorothiazide & hydralazine
Hydromox-R	quinethazone & reserpine
Hydropres	hydrochlorothiazide & reserpine
Inderide	hydrochlorothiazide & propranolol
Maxzide	hydrochlorothiazide & triamterene
Metatensin	trichlormethiazide & reserpine

(continues on next page)

(continued from previous page)

COMBINATION MEDICINES (continued)

Minizide	polythiazide & prazosin
Moduretic	hydrochlorothiazide & amiloride
Naquival	trichlormethiazide & reserpine
Oreticyl	hydrochlorothiazide & reserpine
Oreticyl Forte	hydrochlorothiazide & reserpine
Rauzide	bendroflumethiazide & reserpine
Regroton	chlorthalidone & reserpine
Renese-R	polythiazide & reserpine
Salutensin	hydroflumethiazide & reserpine
Salutensin-Demi	hydroflumethiazide & reserpine
Ser-Ap-Es	hydrochlorothiazide & reserpine & hydralazine
Serpasil-Apresoline	reserpine & hydralazine
Serpasil-Esidrix	hydrochlorothiazide & reserpine
Tenoretic	chlorthalidone & atenolol
Timolide	hydrochlorothiazide & timolol
Tri-Hydroserpine	hydrochlorothiazide & reserpine & hydralazine

NOTES

NOTES

NOTES

NOTES

NOTES

NOTES

NOTES

NOTES

NOTES

NOTES

NOTES

NOTES